The Great Big Fitness Quote Book: <u>Over 365 Motivational Quotes</u> To Help You Get Back In Shape!

Compiled by Cameron M. Clark
Biographical Summaries written by
Cameron M. Clark

Book 1 in 'The Great Big Quote Books'
series

Published by Paul St. George Press

Email: greatbigquotebooks@gmail.com

© 2015

ISBN-13: 978-1523410873

ISBN-10: 1523410876

Preface

I love words. I love the way many words sound. I love the gift of language that we human beings have been given to make it easy in most cases, for us to communicate. Not only that, I love the way we can put words together to mean something. We can tell someone else what we are thinking, feeling or planning to do. Hopefully, you feel the same way about language.

Language is a beautiful thing. But language that can motivate and inspire others is supernal. What greater gift can you give someone than to express to that man, woman or child some form of wisdom, insight or experience that might give them the direction they need to take a positive action that will improve their lives?

It was with the above sentiment that I tried to approach this project. As a regular practitioner of sensible fitness and nutrition for over two decades, I have had a passion for the concept of self-improvement and the desire to move past our previously perceived limits. I have seen it happen in my own life repeatedly and I've seen it in the lives of those around me.

Over the years, in this pursuit of improved health and fitness, I've collected numerous motivational quotes from many successful individuals from all walks of life. I've kept them in notebooks and journals along with applications on my phone and computer. I have a personal library at home that contains dozens of books on health, fitness and nutrition. In addition, I went to the library to do more research on what the latest authorities are publishing in their own books that hasn't been published online yet. It was only recently that I thought of sharing them with you.

You see, this isn't just another fitness quote book where a compiler copied and pasted a bunch of quotes from a bunch of websites and then put it into book form. Why would I do that when there are plenty of people putting books like that on the market?

Instead, I also used quotes from lesser-known, but knowledgable, credible folks like bodybuilding writer and fitness expert Stuart McRobert, strength coach, John Christy and celebrity personal trainer Kathy Kaehler. There are also a few quotes from five-time national bench press champion Brooks Kubik, Olympic gold medal swimmer Dara Torres, former champion bodybuilder Lee Labrada, Bill Baroni and so many more. These are people whose words of wisdom and inspiration were not easily aggregated on the Internet from some website or a couple of websites that specialize in motivational quotes. Instead, I wanted to give something new and original to you, the reader. I can't emphasize my passion for doing this enough. As you go through the book's pages, hopefully you will see that even though these are the words of other individuals, I am trying to communicate something important to you as well.

What you hold in your hands is a book that has collected the words of scores of professional fitness trainers, Olympic athletes, professional athletes, martial artists, old-time strongmen, ancient philosophers, a few motivational experts, professional sports coaches and a couple normal people who knew that achieving their goal of getting into better shape was going to take commitment, determination, willpower and some planning. These are men and women, just like you and me, who face the many challenges of a busy lifestyle that include supporting families, engaging in full-time professions and performing volunteer work. However, these people still have maintained some semblance of health and fitness, knowing how important it all is.

There are over 365 quotations in this book from many people in the above-mentioned fields. I refrained from including too many general motivational quotes that could be applied to any other aspect of life, because I think it is so important to have a context in which the words will make sense. Most of the quotes are meant for inspirational and motivational purposes. There is very little instruction in this book. That was a deliberate choice on my part because I don't know where you might be on this journey to self-improvement.

What's so great about motivational quotations is that they can have the same impact to motivate the amateur powerlifter, the working mother of 3 who wants to get into better shape or the aspiring competitive athlete. It doesn't matter your walk in life as long as you're moving in the direction you want to go.

As I was compiling this book, I came to the realization of how important the mind is in this whole process of "getting and staying in shape." It is amazing how much our thinking, decision-making processes and planning can influence whether we succeed or fail. My hope is that a few, many or even all of the words shared in this book will give your mind the boost it needs to take those next steps to improving your health and your life.

Stay strong, be happy, forgive yourself and others, and remember that the journey to a better 'you' is taken one day at a time.

Best wishes,

Cameron M. Clark
January 2015

Introduction

This book of quotations has been compiled for inspirational and motivational purposes only. There is very little in the way of practical instruction in this book and therefore, I encourage you to seek the help of licensed professionals to assist you in planning your sensible nutrition, fitness and other lifestyle plans. **Also, please consult your doctor before embarking on any type of physical fitness or nutrition plan that modifies your current lifestyle.**

This book has over 365 quotations in it from many athletes, coaches, fitness trainers, celebrities and others who have made fitness an important part of their lives. My intention was that you would have a different quote for each day to carry with you throughout the year. Before beginning this project, I searched for any similar resources on the market to what I had imagined. While I found a number of websites and even some ebooks that were intended for the same purpose as what I set out to do, many only included quotes from motivational experts in business and industry. This book is different in that I really tried to go back to the many quotes I've collected over time that actually had to do with improving oneself in health and fitness.

I took a couple of extra steps in creating something that I really hope will help you.

I organized the quotations into dozens of separate categories. There are those that you would expect like "Nutrition," "Commitment," "Energy" and "Strength." I also wanted to include categories or themes that would be not as obvious, but just as important to overall health such as "Aging," "Discipline," "Focus," "Goal Setting" and "Relaxation" to help you in your search for a specific area of inspiration. My hope is that if you want help in overcoming obstacles or dealing with failure or sticking to a certain eating plan, it will be easier to find the encouraging words you are looking for to get you moving in the right track again by searching categories.

The other step I took was to write brief biographical summaries of all of those people quoted in this book. This was not easy in some cases. You can find these listed in alphabetical order in the back of the book. I don't know about you, but I shudder when I hear a speaker or see a social media personality quote someone of whom they clearly have no knowledge. Even as I was doing my research for this book, I found another motivational book that had quoted a totalitarian dictator who'd oppressed his people during his rule. It was clear that the author had no understanding of what this person had done during his cruel reign.

Quoting a person out of context can seem empty and cause the words to lose their intended impact. My hope is that at least one of those people quoted in this book will be someone you will seek after for more information and want to learn more about their way of doing things.

While these biographical summaries are not extensive or all-inclusive, many of them included 3 categories:

1. 'Occupation' - In some cases, I could have included a dozen occupations, but instead tried to keep it to no more than three.

2. 'Known for' -In most cases, the people I quoted were usually known outside of their own social circles for some accomplishment such as winning a gold medal at the Olympics or appearing as a fitness trainer on television. Whenever I was able to include that information, I did so.

3. 'Published works include' - I restricted these lists to the actual books that were written by the quoted individuals. I thought it was

important to give you a starting point of where you could find more of the writings of these individuals.

Also, if you see an error or would like more information about what I've shared in this book or if you want to be included in future mailings to let you know about other 'Great Big Quote Books' we are planning, feel free to email me at greatbigquotebooks@gmail.com.

This is Book One in 'The Great Big Quote Books' series.

Enjoy!

Invitation

Like the book? I'd love a review! Please feel free to give your feedback on www.Amazon.com to let others know what you thought about this book. As you know, there are some things I really tried to do different with this than a lot of the other quote books you find on Amazon that seem to just be a quick copy-and-paste style collection of quotes.

Also, if you want more information on 'The Great Big Quote Books' series, you can follow us on Instagram: @greatbigquotebooks. You can also 'like' us on Facebook by clicking:

https://www.facebook.com/greatbigquotebooks. We will be posting many quotes on Fitness, Love & Success that you can share with your friends through social media. Also, keep watching for other great deals, such as book giveaways!

'The Great Big Love Quote Book,' 'The Great Big Fitness Quote Book' and 'The Great Big Success Quote Book' are on sale on Amazon.com.

Acknowledgements

I've learned that an essential part of good health, fitness and well-being is the expression of gratitude. I would be remiss if I didn't thank a few people:

My wife, Cara is first on my list for giving me the space and time I needed to complete this project. Whenever someone undertakes a large, creative project, there is likely always an underestimation of how much time and effort it will actually require to complete, but I am happy to say Cara has supported me in every way possible in getting this done. She's also been my proofreader and has done an excellent job. I love her for it.

To my kids, Brinley, Macy and Austin. I love each of them and I appreciate them giving daddy his time and space to get this done as well. My hope for them is that they will continue to live long, happy, healthy and active lives.

My brother, Kenlon, he has been a creative force in his own right and someone who has continually motivated me with his encouragement and belief in me. We send Voxer messages to each other almost daily on our phones and I don't know if I could get things done without that encouragement.

My mom and dad, who have been examples of an active lifestyle and always being on the move. On vacations, we would take a hike in the morning, swim in the afternoon and then find some other active and fun activity at night. My mom says I was exercising with her on the floor of our living room at two years of age.

My sister, Cassell decided to get to a healthy level of fitness and stay there through sensible eating choices and activity. She has shown that no matter what your age and what your circumstances, people can make healthy choices and commitments and then stick with them.

To my sister, Kyla, who has been active her entire life. I believe she may have been the first person who introduced me to weight training and the formal concepts and principles of getting into and staying in shape at the wee age of 10.

To my publisher, Paul St. George Press, I thank them for their assistance in getting this published.

Also, a big 'thank you' to iPriest for helping me format this for Createspace.

And finally a huge "thank you" to those in this book who have gone before and blazed the trail of health and fitness. Their words of inspiration are amazing! Many of these people are giants with a legacy they are building or have left behind, whose only true desire was to help their fellowmen and women. And I want to send out a big "thank you" to all of these pioneers of health and fitness for their words of wisdom.

Action

1. "If you spend too much time thinking about a thing, you'll never get it done. Make at least one definite move daily toward your goal."

- Bruce Lee -

2. "What you feel doesn't matter in the end; it's what you do that makes you brave."

- Andre Agassi -

3. "Standing still is never a good option. Not in the ring, and not in life outside the octagon either. When you stop moving, you're done. When the status quo becomes your main weapon, your arsenal is diminished. When you can find no other way forward except for repetition, your mistakes are compounded into defeat."

- Georges St. Pierre -

4. "Do something, anything, that gets the blood and oxygen pumping, lights up the brain and works the muscles!"

- Bill Phillips -

5. "It takes more effort to wait than to act. Procrastination is tiring and soul-sapping. Waiting for the perfect opportunity is stifling and confining. You can wait for an opportunity, or you can create an opportunity."

- Urijah Faber -

6. "Motivation is the willpower to take action and sustain action on the information that you have."

- Lee Labrada -

7. "You can't wait for opportunity to come to you, because it won't. You've got to go get it. If you don't make things happen, they won't happen."

- Ben Weider -

8. "There's no specific type of body motion that anyone has to do. Any type of body motion performed at the effective level of intensity will cause the release of those good brain chemicals and give you that feeling you're seeking."

- Jay Cooper-

9. "Never put an age limit on your dreams."

- Dara Torres -

10. "The body and mind are one. When the intimate relationship between mind and body is disrupted, aging and entropy accelerate. Restoring mind/body integration brings about renewal. Through conscious breathing and movement techniques, you can renew the body/mind and reverse the aging process."

- Deepak Chopra -

11. "Age is no barrier. It's a limitation you put on your mind."

- Jackie Joyner-Kersee -

12. "There are two things that you have to do in life: you have to die, and you have to live until you die. The rest is up to you."

- Urijah Faber -

13. "Train for health and physique, not just physique. Health comes first. You may not believe it now if you're young, but you will believe it later on when you're not-so-young."

- Stuart McRobert -

14. "Today you may be relatively young, but now is the time to outwit old age."

- Jack LaLanne -

15. "Swimming is a great option for people with arthritis or balance issues that can limit their ability to perform weight-bearing exercise."

- James Beckerman -

16. "You simply cannot escape this reality: Your body is the epicenter of your universe. You go nowhere without it. It is truly the temple of your mind and your soul. If it is sagging, softening, and aging rapidly, other aspects of your life will soon follow suit."

- Bill Phillips -

17. "Your workouts require commitment, determination, planning, consistency, and intensity. If you don't like what you're doing, then there's no way on earth you'll succeed. Enthusiasm is a huge piece of the puzzle. Get creative and stay curious."

- Tony Horton -

18. "Some people die at 25 but aren't buried until they're 75."

- Benjamin Franklin -

19. "Nobody who ever gave his best regretted it."

- George Halas -

20. "It is not the size of a man but the size of his heart that matters."

- Evander Holyfield -

21. "Passion is a huge prerequisite to winning. It makes you willing to jump through hoops, go through all the ups and downs and everything in between to reach your goal."

- Kerri Walsh -

22. "Fight adversity with passion."

- Urijah Faber -

23. "If you always put limits on everything you do, physical or anything else, it will spread into your work and into your life. There are no limits. There are only plateaus, and you must not stay there, you must go beyond them."

- Bruce Lee -

24. "You have far more control over your own life and destiny than you probably give yourself credit for. Grab this control, and get doing what you know you need to be doing. There is so much more you can do with your life to make it more rewarding and enjoyable, if only you would challenge yourself to do more with it, and stop procrastinating well-planned action."

- Stuart McRobert -

25. "When I pass on to that great gym in the sky I want no more than for people to say: 'He was marvelously alive!'"

- Jack LaLanne -

26. "To be successful, you must dedicate yourself 100% to your training, diet and mental approach."

- Arnold Schwarzenegger -

27. "Fitness isn't just the goal – it's a lifestyle that will allow you to look and feel your best, and in turn, to live your best life."

- Kathy Kaehler -

28. "Pull yourself together. Employ self-fulfilling body language. Stand up straight. Shoulders back. Chest out. Chin up. Carry yourself young. Defy gravity. Believe in the self-fulfilling prophecy – a youthful posture will support youthful self-imagery and attitude. It is subtle but effective."

- Walter M. Boortz II -

29. "Building a body is no different from how you would approach any other building project. You must first have a vision of what you want to build, of what exactly you are looking to do. Don't cheat yourself. Go for it all."

- Steve Michalik –

30. "I try to come at fitness and nutrition from a perspective of gentleness and what will make me feel good afterwards. I try to stay out of the mindset of needing to fix myself. I do whatever seems fun to me."

- Taylor Schilling -

31. "Look for ways to recover better between workouts, like making sure that your caloric intake is where is should be. Look for ways to concentrate better during your workouts so you can train harder and with better form."

- John Christy -

32. "Open your mind to the possibility that your body is incredible and capable of amazing things. This might be hard to do, especially if you're used to putting yourself down or entertaining negative thoughts about yourself. But know this: There is nothing wrong or horrible about who you are. You and your body are unique and amazing!"

- Kim Lyons -

33. "What is the ultimate purpose of your life? What is it you feel, in your heart, that you're meant to accomplish in the time you're here?"

- Bill Phillips -

34. "When you say yes to taking time for yourself, you are honoring your need to play as well as to work, whether you're a stay-at-home mom or a jet-setting businesswoman."

- Denise Austin -

35. "A youthful mind is dynamic, vibrant, and curious. This is what we all desire - an alert vibrant mind along with strong physical vitality."

- Deepak Chopra -

36. "Whatever you believe about dieting, you're probably right. Whatever you believe about your abilities, your good luck or misfortune, your opportunities, the condition of your relationships, you're probably right!"

- Chalene Johnson -

Balance

37. "One of the most important things you can do if you hope to reach your goals is to give yourself some freedom to occasionally eat unwisely. What's key, though, is that after it happens you then let it go. Move on. No one ever did a tremendous amount of damage to him- or herself at one meal, let alone in one day."

- Bob Greene -

38. "Be obsessed, focused and consumed by your training when you are in the gym, and rest, eat and sleep well while out of the gym. Then get on with the rest of your life."

- Stuart McRobert -

39. "I'm tired of reading books on powerlifting. I want to read good literature. I want to travel. To see things, go to museums, do things that make me happy."

- Joe Weider –

40. "Regularity in the hours of rising and retiring, perseverance in exercise, adaptation of dress to the variations of climate, simple and nutritious aliment, and temperance in all things are necessary branches of the regimen of health."

- Philip Stanhope -

41. "I like to embrace natural beauty. I try to get at least 8 hours of sleep, drinking a lot of water and exercising."

- Tia Mowry -

42. "Maintaining your ideal weight is a physical sign that you are in balance. Feeling contented and fulfilled shows that your mind and emotions have found balance."

- Deepak Chopra -

43. "Getting fit is all about reaching for, achieving, and sustaining a commitment to taking care of yourself for the rest of your life. You might need to make adaptations – to keep feeding surprises to your body and mind just to keep things fun. But change does not mean stopping or giving up."

- Dara Torres -

44. "The most common question I am asked is: 'Jack, how do you do it? How do you keep up the pace of daily workouts and eating only the healthiest of foods? Don't you ever get tempted to fall off the wagon?' My answer to them is: 'You bet I do! But I don't do it!'"

- Jack LaLanne -

45. "There are only two options regarding commitment; you're either in or you're out. There's no such thing as life in-between."

- Pat Riley -

46. "If you aren't going all the way, why go at all?"

- Joe Namath -

47. "Start the year off right and make a commitment to making it the best training year that you've ever had."

- John Christy -

48. "Traumatic experiences challenge us. They challenge our lifestyle commitments but they don't spell complete disaster. Nothing ever does that, because our lifestyles never end."

- Bill Baroni -

49. "By following through on your daily health commitments, you grow your own self-worth so that you can take greater and greater control of your machine. As this happens, you begin to see your potential to take on bigger challenges. Your machine is at your command. You start to see that your target is within reach."

- Chris Powell -

50. "A big reason why so many people have trouble staying on track is that they get caught up in the latest trend and don't focus on what they need as individuals."

- Tony Horton -

51. "You can always improve your fitness if you keep training."

- Pastor Maldonado -

52. "Change must come gradually, and it must come as a result of the realistic incorporation of healthy habits into your daily lifestyle."

- Tony Horton -

53. "We are what we repeatedly do. Excellence, therefore, is not an act, but a habit."

- Aristotle -

54. "I love habits! Having a collection of good habits is like being the head of a company of highly skilled employees who do their jobs without needing constant management. The company runs itself, leaving you free to make the big decisions."

- Leslie Sansone -

55. "Success isn't always about 'greatness.' It's about consistency. Consistent, hard work gains success. Greatness will come."

- Dwayne Johnson -

56. "It's the little details that are vital. Little things make big things happen."

- John Wooden -

57. "I fear not the man who has practiced 10,000 kicks once, but I fear the man who has practiced one kick 10,000 times."

- Bruce Lee -

58. "The ingredients to lasting success in any area are universal, and one of the key ingredients is our consistent action. Those actions become our habits. Those habits change our thinking. Those habits change our body. Those habits define our destiny."

- Chalene Johnson -

59. "The most successful business travelers keep their daily schedules as consistent as possible, whether at home or in a foreign country. This means waking up and going to bed at similar times, exercising at a similar intensity and time of day, and maintaining similar eating habits."

- Chris Carmichael -

60. "Consistency is the key to changing a negative habit. You must make the commitment to do something about your shape and your physical condition each and every day, day after day, week after week, month after month."

- Lee Labrada -

61. "Get fit. Stay fit. Live fit. Do those three things, and you'll reach your ultimate destination: Pants fit."

- David Zinczenko -

62. "It's not about how many times you fall down, but how many times you get back up."

- Abraham Lincoln -

63. "I'm scared of failure all the time but I'm not scared enough to stop trying."

- Ronda Rousey -

64. "When we go off course we need to identify it, correct it, accept it, forgive ourselves and move on. We don't need to try to make up for overeating one day by starving the next. Just put it behind you and get back to your healthy nutrition plan the following day."

- Bill Phillips -

65. "Some people learn to lose. Others lose and learn."

- Georges St. Pierre -

66. "Even if you fall on your face, you're still moving forward."

- Victor Kiam -

67. "There is no failure except in no longer trying."

- Elbert Hubbard -

68. "Defeat is a state of mind; no one is ever defeated until defeat has been accepted as a reality."

- Bruce Lee -

69. "It is a rough road that leads to the heights of greatness."

- Seneca the Younger -

70. "I've missed more than 9,000 shots in my career. I've lost almost 300 games. Twenty six times I've been trusted to take the game winning shot and missed. I've failed over and over and over again in my life. And that is why I succeed."

- Michael Jordan -

71. "Anytime you undertake any difficult task, you have to face the possibility of short-term failure, obstacles that block your path and have to be overcome. Failure doesn't have to discourage you. It can be a great training tool."

- Arnold Schwarzenegger -

72. "Forget mistakes. Forget failure. Forget everything except what you're going to do now and do it. Today is your lucky day."

- Will Durant -

73. "Failing is not a terminal condition. It's a process. How we interpret failures and act upon them ultimately determines whether we persist in, and exist in, failure. Or overcome our temporary obstacles to become a success."

- Lee Labrada -

74. "If you're not making mistakes, then you're not doing anything. I'm positive that a doer makes mistakes."

- John Wooden -

75. "There is no such thing as a lost cause, or a dead end. Through persistence, attitude, and creativity, there's always an escape route."

- Urijah Faber -

Determination

76. "When life puts you in tough situations. Don't say 'why me,' just say 'try me.'"

- Dwayne Johnson -

77. "Either I will find a way, or I will make one."

- Phillip Sidney -

78. "The price of success is hard work, dedication to the job at hand, and the determination that whether we win or lose, we have applied the best of ourselves to the task at hand."

- Vince Lombardi -

79. "The five S's of sports training are: stamina, speed, strength, skill, and spirit; but the greatest of these is spirit."

- Ken Doherty -

80. "When animals surrender they go lying on their back. I never go lying on my back. It's a sign of weakness and surrendering. Never lying on my back."

- Mikko Salo -

81. "We all have dreams. But in order to make dreams come into reality, it takes an awful lot of determination, dedication, self-discipline, and effort."

- Jesse Owens -

82. "Keep following your heart and you'll just fall into the life you were meant to lead. And be confident because everybody around is going to tell you 'no.'"

- Gina Carano -

83. "This ability to conquer oneself is no doubt the most precious of all things sports bestows."

- Olga Korbut -

84. "All successes begin with self-discipline. It starts with you."

- Dwayne Johnson-

85. "Without self-discipline, success is impossible, period."

- Lou Holtz -

86. "Conquer yourself, and the world lives at your feet."

- St. Augustine -

87. "What makes something special is not just what you have to gain, but what you feel there is to lose."

- Andre Agassi -

88. "With discipline, belief, and the right knowledge, we become the best we can be."

- Georges St. Pierre -

89. "Rather than finding reasons why something cannot be done, though you know it needs to be done, get on with doing it. See problems as challenges. And apply such an attitude change throughout your life – not just to training-related matters – and then delight in seeing your life change for the better."

- Stuart McRobert -

90. "People embark on a get in shape program with the intention of changing for the better, but fail for two reasons: they lack the correct information, and they are unable to get motivated and stay motivated."

- Lee Labrada -

91. "There are no guarantees in this life, but we can live our days with healthy activities to get as near to perfect health, fitness and physique as possible."

- Jack LaLanne -

92. "Constantly see yourself in your mind's eye doing more than you currently do."

- Bradley J. Steiner -

93. "Our choices should typically be guided by what's right, not necessarily by what's easiest, most comfortable, or most convenient. That's really what self-discipline is all about."

- Tony Horton -

94. "Once you understand the concept of taking responsibility for your life, it's time to move on to knowing what you really want – regarding your body, mind, and soul!"

- Bob Greene -

95. "If a man achieves victory over this body, who in the world can exercise power over him? He who rules himself rules over the whole world."

- Vinoba Bhave -

96. "The space between hunger and eating, where you make the choice you want to make, isn't empty. It is filled with awareness. Awareness is close to what people call an open mind. You're free to think the thoughts you want to have."

- Deepak Chopra -

97. "You can outsmart the supermarket to make healthy choices... When you walk into the store, head directly to the produce – it is typically on the side of the store near the entrance. It is close to the door because produce is profitable, so use this to your advantage and stock up there first. Do not be distracted by other items – salad dressings and baked goods can sometimes sneak their way into this area."

- James Beckerman -

98. "If you are going to win any battle you have to do one thing. You have to make the mind run the body. Never let the body tell the mind what to do. The body will always give up. It is always tired in the morning, noon and night. But the body is never tired if the mind is not tired."

- George S. Patton -

Education

99. "Seek out information from reliable sources that have a proven track record. And always look for evidence, facts, and testimonials that back up and validate the credibility of that information."

- Jillian Michaels -

100. "Focus, discipline, hard work, goal setting and, of course, the thrill of finally achieving your goals. These are all lessons in life."

- Kristi Yamaguchi -

101. "Knowing is not enough, we must apply. Willing is not enough, we must do."

- Bruce Lee -

102. "Wisdom is always an overmatch for strength."

- Phil Jackson -

103. "Today is the start of the rest of your life. You will never be as young as you are now. Learn from your mistakes and those of others, get in charge of your own destiny, and make the most of the now – make each day count."

- Stuart McRobert -

104. "I keep the white-belt mentality that I can learn from anyone, anywhere, anytime."

- Georges St. Pierre -

105. "Nothing beats solid, sensible nutrition and regular exercise when it comes to losing weight and keeping it off, no matter what the ads say!"

- Kim Lyons -

106. "Physical care of your body isn't enough. If you live with resentment, anger, or other destructive emotions, you'll tear yourself apart from within. Happiness is an essential part of good health."

- Stuart McRobert -

107. "Men are like steel. When they lose their temper, they lose their worth."

- Chuck Norris -

108. "The Iron is the best antidepressant I have ever found. There is no better way to fight weakness than with strength. Once the mind and body have been awakened to their true potential, it's impossible to turn back."

- Henry Rollins -

109. "Letting go of repressed anger and resentments through courageous and bold acts of forgiveness helps us begin to heal emotionally. This is vitally important because in a very real way, our bodies and lives tend to reflect our inner-emotional condition."

- Bill Phillips -

110. "The accumulation of toxins in the body/mind system accelerates aging. Elimination of toxins awakens the capacity for renewal. Toxins must be identified and eliminated from your body, mind, and soul."

- Deepak Chopra -

Endurance

111. "Most people never run far enough on their first wind to find out they've got a second."

- William James -

112. "It's not whether you get knocked down; it's whether you get up."

- Vince Lombardi -

113. "When the going gets tough, it is always the mind that fails first, not the body."

- Arnold Schwarzenegger -

114. "The true holistic approach to developing more endurance is one in which all aspects of the athlete are considered—these are the triad of structural, chemical, and mental fitness and health."

- Philip Maffetone -

115. "Exercise actually creates time, because it adds longevity. If you invest 30 minutes in yourself each day, you can keep yourself full of energy well into your golden years."

- Lee Labrada -

116. "Training stimulates muscle growth. But for your training to work, your body needs a sufficient amount of energy and enough raw materials to get the full benefit from your exercise program. Providing the energy and those raw materials is the role of nutrition."

- Arnold Schwarzenegger -

117. "Good posture is needed for proper balance and is a prerequisite for a healthy body. Also, the person who carries him or herself with a proud upright posture is more likely to come across as a fit, energetic, desirable individual."

- Jack LaLanne -

118. "Our bodies were designed to generate their own energy, and maintain it at a consistent level. If you're in good health, you should expect to live your whole life in a state of positive energy."

- Denise Austin -

119. "Life is energy. Life consumes energy. All matter is made of energy. It stands to reason that you should learn how to control the energy that runs the mind, body, and life."

- Steve Michalik -

120. "Soon after you begin exercising regularly, you will start to feel better physically and mentally. You will also get subtle signs that your metabolism is changing. Your clothes become looser, and you will have more energy throughout the day."

- Bob Greene -

Enjoyment

121. "Wish not so much to live young, as to live well."

- Benjamin Franklin -

122. "There's a lot of people in this world who spend so much time watching their health that they haven't the time to enjoy it."

- Josh Billings -

123. "A swirl of happiness, enjoyment, and delight, pleasure is an essential part of a happy life."

- Denise Austin -

124. "I'm not exaggerating when I say that when I built up my health with proper exercise and superior nutrition, every day was a joy. I mean it. Every day. And it's still that way. Sure I'm going to die one day. That happens to all of us. But isn't it exciting to know we can push the barriers and regain the health, strength and energy of our younger years?"

- Jack LaLanne -

125. "Several studies show that people tend to remember the peaks and ends of any experience. So try to focus on a peak moment during your last workout, perhaps when you had a real rush of energy. Also consider the sense of gratification you had when you finished."

- Tom Rath -

126. "It is an indispensable requisite before any practical and permanent benefit can be derived from exercise, that it should be attractive and enjoyable. Any form of exercise that may be found so attractive as to be persistently followed up, merits consideration."

- Eugene Sandow -

127. "I am a firm believer in rewarding yourself for the hard work it takes to change lifelong behaviors, and sometimes this involves food. Maybe that means having an extravagant meal or a wonderful dessert now and again."

- Bob Greene -

128. "A trophy carries dust. Memories last forever."

- Mary Lou Retton –

129. "Fitness needs to be perceived as fun and games or we subconsciously avoid it."

- Alan Thicke -

130. "These days, I'm not working out to lose weight. I'm not even working out to maintain my weight. I do it because I love how it feels. I love the energy. The endorphins. The rush. I do it because I learned to trade in the fake rush of donuts and junk food for something more exhilarating: a healthy lifestyle."

- Bill Baroni -

131. "And in the end it's not the years in your life that count. It's the life in your years."

- Abraham Lincoln -

132. "We all need some excitement in our lives. When it comes to working out, we tend to appreciate familiarity and remain loyal to what works for us, but it's important to venture outside of our comfort zones and try different things that offer different benefits. The same principle applies to our relationships, work situations, and other choices in life."

- Tony Horton -

133. "Living the dream is simply a form of living out your passion, of making that passion gradually, through persistence and effort, a central part of your life."

- Urijah Faber -

134. "Remember, what you see in the mirror is far less important than how you feel deep inside. Being happy from within gives you a glow that can't be beat!"

- Kathy Kaehler -

135. "Wake up determined. Go to bed satisfied."

- Dwayne Johnson -

136. "Always make a total effort, even when the odds are against you."

- Arnold Palmer -

137. "Exercise can be used like a vaccine to prevent disease and a medication to treat it. If there were a drug with the same benefits as working out, it would instantly be the standard of care."

- Robert Sallis -

138. "Exercise could almost be called nature's cure-all. It's amazing in its powers. Exercise helps to increase your energy, it cleans out your arteries, improves your posture, increases your mobility, adds muscle and tone, improves strength, builds confidence, burns fat, strengthens bones, hypes your metabolism, augments your flexibility, strengthens your immune system, and shapes your body like nothing else in the world."

- Jack LaLanne -

139. "Exercise is the spark. Nutrition is the fuel. Without both, there can be no flame – no results."

- Bill Phillips –

140. "I encourage you to move your body most days. Doing so will help you avoid what I call exercise bipolar disorder, or EBD. When you exercise, your brain increases the output of feel-good chemicals like dopamine, norepinephrine, serotonin, and adrenaline."

- Tony Horton -

141. "For many people, exercise means an uncomfortable, regimented routine of difficult activities that make us sweat and grunt. Yet the truth is, exercise is nothing more than intentional body motion."

- Jay Cooper -

142. "It's astounding what exercise can do for you. Sure, it makes you stronger and beautifully sculpts your body, but there's a whole lot more to it. Exercise delivers nutrients to all of your cells and oxygenates your organs, tissues, and muscles, giving you tons of energy."

- Chris Powell -

143. "Tell me the last time you went for a walk, hike, or bike ride and felt really bad afterward. Tell me the last time you came home from exercising and said, 'Gee, I'm really sorry I did that.' It doesn't work that way. You always feel good after exercising."

- Leslie Sansone -

144. "Warm up before stretching. Muscles are like taffy: Try to stretch them when they are cold, and they'll snap! Stretch them when they are warm and they'll elongate easily."

- Kim Lyons -

145. "Exercise is an important part of the foundation upon which to build healthy eating habits."

- Bob Greene -

146. "Cardio is great for your heart, but so is resistance training. And unlike cardio, resistance training can kick your metabolism into high gear, helping you burn fat like there's no tomorrow. Cardio work alone just isn't enough."

- Lee Labrada -

147. "Fad diets are nothing more than bogus schemes designed to cause dramatic and rapid weight loss for desperate dieters. They are monotonous, unrealistic, and restrictive and only teach you how to set outrageous boundaries on your eating."

- Kim Lyons -

148. "If it sounds too good to be true, it's probably not worth your time or your dime. Stay away from programs that promise unrealistic results; promote the idea of super fast weight loss; require you to purchase special products, supplements, or foods; or include claims that a certain elixir wipes out diseases."

- Tony Horton -

149. "There is nothing so wearisome as having to be extremely particular about what one eats or drinks. I can never believe that the food faddist is happy."

- Thomas Inch -

150. "One of the most important things you can do for your health is eat of varied diet. Because each food you eat contains a unique assortment of nutrients, the more diverse your diet, the more diverse the nutrients you'll end up getting. Variety keeps eating interesting, too. Your meals are likely to be more satisfying if you haven't eaten the same thing the day before."

- Bob Greene -

151. "You have to turn your back on all of the popular follies and mass-marketed delusions that have shaped you to the present. You have to begin to create a new person – A new self – a new you!"

- Brooks Kubik -

152. "Forget all the pills. The magic shakes. The celebrity exercise DVDs. This is the hard way, the only way, the way that really works. Lifestyle change is not just for a couple of months. It's for the rest of your life."

- Bill Baroni -

153. "People are not overweight – they are over fat. Throw away your scales because weight is irrelevant. It is not your body weight that matters, it's your body fat you should be concerned with."

- Steve Michalik -

154. "Weight loss is a game of calories in versus calories out, and the only way to expend calories and burn off true fat is with a balanced nutrition formula and regular exercise plan."

- Kim Lyons -

155. "The only way to lose weight is to burn more calories a day than you eat!"

- Leslie Sansone -

Flexibility

156. "Flexibility is crucial to my fitness. Incorporating a good warm-up and cool-down into every session decreases my chances of injury. I use both dynamic and static stretching in my training. I've starting doing a few yoga sessions which incorporates muscle strength and flexibility."

- Samantha Stosur -

157. "Being flexible – and doing the work that builds flexibility – also increases strength. Flexibility seems to enhance the muscles' responsiveness, making them more receptive to strength stimuli like resistance training."

- Tony Horton -

158. "Flexibility is probably the most overlooked aspect of fitness, but while it's less glamorous than cardio and strength training, it is no less important."

- Kim Lyons -

159. "Flexibility is the key to stability."

- John Wooden -

160. "Stretching is important for people at any age but especially once we pass 30. As we age, our bodies naturally tighten up – or joints become less mobile... and our muscles stay in a contractive position for long periods... which leads them to atrophy."

- Dara Torres -

161. "When it comes to flexibility, don't assume more is better. There is a consensus among many health care professionals that the least flexible and the most flexible individuals are more likely to get injured compared to those whose joints had moderate flexibility."

- Philip Maffetone -

162. "Flexibility is crucial for preventing injuries and staying mobile. By stretching regularly you can keep your muscles limber, increase your range of motion, improve your balance, and enhance your posture."

- Kathy Kaehler -

163. "A muscle is like a car. If you want it to run well early in the morning, you have to warm it up."

- Florence Griffith Joyner -

164. "Success at anything will always come down to this: focus and effort and we control both."

- Dwayne Johnson -

165. "Let go of any belief you might have that labels your fitness as sacrifice. That's focusing on the things that you've lost. Focus instead on what you have gained, and will always continue to gain by following your new lifestyle."

- Bill Baroni -

166. "I used to think that showing up every day to work out was enough. It isn't. It's what you do and how hard you do it that makes the difference between losing weight and not. Working in the zone is the key to success."

- Oprah Winfrey -

167. "Concentrate your mind up on the idea of acquiring health and strength."

- George Hackenschmidt -

168. "Get each day right, each workout right, and each week right, and then you will get the months right."

- Stuart McRobert -

169. "The ability to concentrate begins with the formation of clearly defined training goals. You must determine exactly what it is that you wish to achieve from your training. Your goals should be stated as clearly and effectively as possible."

- Brooks Kubik -

170. "We always tend to get more of what we focus on in life. It's true. This means it's vitally important to be mindful of where our attention is."

- Bill Phillips -

171. "You can make it to the top without a lot of things – but there never yet was a man who made it without the resolve to do so!"

- Bradley J. Steiner -

172. "What you habitually think largely determines what you will ultimately become."

- Bruce Lee -

173. "Pampering yourself and rewarding yourself through nurturing incentives can go a long way in helping you achieve not only your goals but also fulfillment in your life overall."

- Jillian Michaels -

174. "The scariest thing is setting your goals too low and meeting them."

- Georges St. Pierre -

175. "Set your goals high, and don't stop till you get there."

- Bo Jackson -

176. "Gauge your long-term goals on the basis of what is realistic for most typical people to train with weights, provided they can give their pound of flesh and deliver the dedication, determination, effort and persistence that are needed."

- Stuart McRobert -

177. "When you begin to focus on making progress, one day at a time, towards your goals, you'll discover that you don't have to wait 12 or 18 weeks to really start feeling good about yourself. You can do it every day, starting now."

- Bill Phillips -

178. "By identifying your goals and keeping them clear in your mind, you strengthen your chances of accomplishing them. But remember to listen to your body. Once you begin working out, your body will tell you how it feels, but it's up to you to pay attention and respect the message."

- Dara Torres -

179. "Whatever your goal in life, whether it's to have a world-class physique, or to obtain your own personal fitness goals, it is a game, as all of life is a game. The body and the mind are two players in this game. Sometimes they work together, sometimes they oppose each other. The body will oppose vigorously any changes made to it's structure. Only through the force and the power of the mind can you overcome this resistance. You are your weakest link!"

- Steve Michalik -

180. "Journals are a great way to stay on track with a fitness program. They keep you accountable to yourself and your goals, and serve as a recorded measure of your successes, setbacks, and ultimate progress."

- Kim Lyons -

181. "Once you get hooked on being fit, you maybe come to find that the best reward you can give yourself is sticking to your goals!"

- Bill Baroni -

182. "We all need to accept and love ourselves, no matter how we look. That means loving ourselves just as much now as when we reach our goal."

- Bob Greene -

Health

183. "I think it's more important to be fit so that you can be healthy and enjoy activities than it is to have a good body."

- Rachel Blanchard -

184. "There is much more to looking good and feeling great than having big and strong muscles. If you are not healthy on the inside, then sooner or later you will be unable to maintain size and strength on the outside. Your health is of supreme importance."

- Stuart McRobert -

185. "There is no wealth like health."

- Jack LaLanne -

186. "Stick with the basics. Regardless of their goals, everyone needs to take care of their health first. To do this you need to get stronger, get your heart and lungs in good shape, develop a good level of mobility around all major joints, and eat a healthy diet."

- John Christy -

187. "Our growing softness, our increasing lack of physical fitness, is a menace to our security."

- John F. Kennedy -

188. "To have a functioning body and not to use it is like having 20/20 vision and never opening your eyes."

- Bill Phillips -

189. "If we could give every individual the right amount of nourishment and exercise, not too little and not too much, we would have found the safest way to health."

- Hippocrates -

190. "Take care of your body. It's the only place you have to live."

- Jim Rohn -

191. "The way you think, the way you behave, the way you eat, can influence your life by 30 to 50 years."

- Deepak Chopra -

192. "Exercise dramatically enhances your confidence in a number of ways. It makes you feel better about how you look; it releases mood-boosting chemicals in the brain, making you feel better about life in general; and it makes a statement, to yourself and the world, that you are worth taking good care of. Ultimately, when you feel strong physically, you feel strong in other aspects of your life as well."

- Jillian Michaels -

193. "Having strong and fit muscles keeps you looking and feeling good. It increases your ability to play sports, even if you are only a weekend athlete."

- Arnold Schwarzenegger -

194. "No matter who you are, in order to stay young and healthy, you need to move your body. It's as simple as that. Almost every system in your body, from your cardiovascular system to your muscular and skeletal systems, benefits from regular physical activity."

- Kathy Kaehler -

195. "I know a lot of people say: 'If I had the money then I'd be able to achieve health, fitness, peace of mind and joy.' I can't say it enough times: your health account and your bank account are synonymous. The more you put in, the more you can take out. You can't buy health and you can't buy fitness."

- Jack Lalanne -

196. "This is what fitness really boils down to: feeling good inside your skin and in your clothes, trusting that you can get out of bed with a spring in your step, and enjoying an active, fun-filled life."

- Dara Torres -

197. "I think fitness is important. I think a healthy lifestyle is important. I think putting positive energy out there is important and just staying connected with the people."

- LL Cool J -

198. "You need to eat normally and healthfully, and you need to exercise. I'm so passionate about this because I think people spend their lives not happy in their bodies."

- Courtney Thorne-Smith -

199. "Getting fit for the rest of your life isn't an act of magic. Anyone can learn how to do it. The skills required are easily taught and easily learned, as well. Just about anyone can put them into practice, and fast. In fact, you can start today."

- Bill Baroni -

200. "Developing a diet that is healthful, balanced, and appropriate for your particular caloric needs is easy enough and is absolutely critical to establishing a healthful lifestyle that incorporates proper nutrition, adequate fitness, and mental resilience."

- Daphne Oz -

201. "People need to know that fitness is not a dimension on the outside, whether your goal is 36-24-36 or whatever. Fitness really is how you feel about yourself internally and your heart space; are you happy internally."

- Cory Everson -

202. "You can reverse your biological age by enhancing the integration between your mind and your body. Mind and body are intimately interconnected."

- Deepak Chopra -

203. "True enjoyment comes from activity of the mind and exercise of the body; the two are ever united."

- Wilhelm von Humboldt -

204. "Physical fitness is not only one of the most important keys to a healthy body, it is the basis of dynamic and creative intellectual activity."

- John F. Kennedy -

205. "Intellectual growth should commence at birth and cease only at death."

- Albert Einstein -

206. "People think athleticism is just physical, but it's not. It's connected to the brain and how the brain can learn to execute and see a movement or not. Especially at high speed. Being athletic is not just jumping and running and being powerful. It's the nervous system that guides the body. The muscles don't decide anything. The brain decides and makes things happen."

- Georges St. Pierre -

207. "Draw motivation from elite–level accomplishments, but get your feet firmly back to earth when it comes to designing your own training program. If you do not do this you will be bang on course for treading the same road to training ruin that millions have already travelled."

- Stuart McRobert -

208. "If you want to learn to swim, jump into the water. On dry land no frame of mind is ever going to help you."

- Bruce Lee -

209. "Motivation is a very personal thing, and what motivates one person might not do it for another. The trick is to find what motivates you personally, and run with it!"

- Kim Lyons -

210. "To succeed…You need to find something to hold on to, something to motivate you, something to inspire you."

- Tony Dorsett -

211. "Knowing that good nutrition will give you the strength and stamina you need to perform your workouts properly it's going to make you want to eat well. You'll become much more conscious of what you're consuming."

- Bob Greene -

212. "Set yourself a goal of a completely pure diet, and then go forward with enthusiasm. Don't change your life out of anxiety. Purity is a positive theme that is meant to increase your sense of joyful living."

- Deepak Chopra -

213. "Bust out of that prison of shame and guilt – the one you built! You're a winner. From this day forward, success is your only option. It's the only choice you have."

- Chalene Johnson -

214. "Fights aren't won in the octagon, they're won in the months leading up to them, in a near-empty gym, in the lost hours of the day, whether I feel like it or not."

- Georges St. Pierre -

215. "I have never gone to the gym just to lose weight. I go to the gym to get and stay healthy, which is vastly more important to me. Being healthy means that you get to enjoy your life. Your friends. Your job. New people. New adventures. Yes, a by-product of feeling healthy is that your weight comes off and stays off. But it also means a smile on your face."

- Bill Baroni -

216. "I can accept failure, everyone fails at something. I can't accept not trying."

- Michael Jordan -

217. "Your biggest opponent isn't the other guy. It's human nature."

- Bobby Knight -

218. "To make healthy eating come naturally, we need to reset our palates back to a state of nature, to relearn the art of savoring food for its built-in flavor."

- Leslie Sansone -

219. "Read labels and look for things made with real food instead of highly processed ingredients. Compare nutrition facts labels to find options that are lower in sodium and sugar and higher in fiber. Just remember that chips, crackers, cookies, ice cream, and other snacks and treats are still extras – even if they are made with green tea or goji berries or air dried sea salt."

- Monica Reinagel -

220. "Every one should and can find out which diet best suits his constitution, and he should avoid all food which disagrees with it."

- George Hackenschimdt -

221. "Please do yourself a favor and commit to eating your vegetables. Stretch outside of your comfort zone and try new ones as often as you can. You'll be surprised by the range of flavors, textures, and colors you will come to love."

- Bob Harper -

222. "What you eat is also important, along with how much. The more you restrict your calories, the more certain you have to be that you're getting the most nutritional density possible – the most bang for your buck."

- Arnold Schwarzenegger -

223. "What you eat today will be walking and talking tomorrow."

- Jack LaLanne -

224. "What you eat has a direct effect on how you feel and how you look. Unhealthy processed foods tax our immune systems and organs, energy, and speed up the aging process. By contrast, healthy, whole foods fuel and heal us in a way that allows our bodies and our minds to do what we ask of them."

- Tony Horton -

225. "Food is the foundation of everything you do. Without the right fats for the aerobic system, energy will be limited. Without the thousands of nutrients from fresh vegetables and fruits, the immune system can't stop the process of illness and disease. And without the balance of macronutrients - the proper amounts of carbohydrates, fats, and proteins your particular body needs - the brain can't continue to thrive."

- Philip Maffetone -

226. "It's extremely important to find out how many calories you're eating because most people underestimate. That's one of the reasons why they aren't getting results and why they put weight in the first place."

- Craig Ballantyne -

227. "Much of your weight-loss battle will go down in the kitchen!"

- Kim Lyons -

228. "The more understanding and clarity people have about how to eat right, the better and faster they can both let go of unhealthy body weight and increase their energy, vitality and well-being."

- Bill Phillips -

229. "When you expect to be tempted with bad choices, try priming before a meal with healthy alternatives. Find something healthy to fill your stomach a little and decrease your appetite."

- Tom Rath -

230. "Human beings were meant to eat a variety of foods. If our bodies were designed to operate like well-run machines on vitamin C alone, we could live happily on a grapefruit diet."

- Bob Greene -

231. "If it has a cartoon character on the box, you should not be eating what is inside."

- James Beckerman -

232. "Nutrition and exercise are like the two wheels of a bicycle: if both are in good working order, the bike will take you anywhere you want to go. However, if one or the other is out of commission, you'll be stuck on your front porch. It's the same with your body."

- Lee Labrada -

233. "Ah, the word 'diet.' It probably makes you think of restriction, deprivation, and boredom, among other disagreeable things. I want you to rethink this four letter word. The word diet simply refers to a pattern of eating. That's it!"

- Chris Powell -

234. "If you stumble once in a while, just put it behind you and resolve to do better from that point forward. The mere fact that you have decided to improve yourself is something to be proud of. Focus on that."

- Bill Phillips -

235. "Obstacles don't have to stop you. If you run into a wall, don't turn around and give up. Figure out how to climb it, go through it or work around it."

- Michael Jordan -

236. "Accept the challenges so that you can feel the exhilaration of victory."

- George S. Patton -

237. "No one will hit you harder than life itself. It doesn't matter how you hit back. It's about how much you can take, and keep fighting, how much you can suffer and keep moving forward. That's how you win."

- Anderson Silva -

238. "The harder the conflict, the more glorious the triumph."

- Thomas Paine -

239. "Making the most of your life is not about earth-shaking achievements. It is about doing your best to be your best. This is not measured merely in terms of what you actually achieve, but by the obstacles you overcame whilst striving to succeed."

- Stuart McRobert -

240. "We have not journeyed across the centuries, across the oceans, across the mountains, across the prairies because we are made of sugar candy."

- Winston Churchill -

241. "I've always found that anything worth achieving will always have obstacles in the way and you've got to have that drive and determination to overcome those obstacles on route to whatever it is that you want to accomplish."

- Chuck Norris -

242. "Adversity causes some men to break; others to break records."

- William A. Ward -

243. "Anytime you try to break out of an old habit, there's a certain amount of negative tension that tries to pull you back toward that old habit. That's because your mind is like a cranky grandfather: it has an internal resistance to change."

- Lee Labrada -

244. "The wall! Your success is on the other side. Can't jump over it or go around it. You know what to do."

- Dwayne Johnson -

245. "Aim to be all that you can be. Carry the hard lessons of self-conquest and discipline that you learn in your training into every facet of your life."

- Bradley J. Steiner -

246. "I firmly believe that any man's finest hour, the greatest fulfillment of all that he holds dear, is that moment when he has worked his heart out in a good cause and lies exhausted on the field of battle – victorious."

- Vince Lombardi -

Patience

247. "Exercise to stimulate, not to annihilate. The world wasn't formed in a day, and neither were we. Set small goals and build upon them."

- Lee Haney -

248. "Fitness is a curve. You can be Lance Armstrong, or you can be really out of shape at the opposite end. People enter the curve wherever they are and then they can move up the curve, by better nutrition and better exercise."

- Gordon Strachan -

249. "Eventually, small goals build up to bigger goals. Which in turn build up to bigger goals. It's a question of degrees, and it only becomes a problem when we set big goals and insist that we get to them now."

- Bill Baroni -

250. "The strongest of all warriors are these two: Time and Patience."

- Leo Tolstoy -

251. "Courage, sacrifice, determination, commitment, toughness, heart, talent, guts. That's what little girls are made of; the heck with sugar and spice."

- Bethany Hamilton -

252. "A lot of people give up just before they're about to make it. You never know when that next obstacle is going to be the last one."

- Chuck Norris -

253. "Persistence is the watch word. No matter what, keep at your training."

- Bradley J. Steiner -

254. "With resistance training and life, the simple, inescapable fact is that maximum intensity occurs after you have 'perceived' failure. Those who can go beyond that – to a higher point – to push themselves to a place where they have not been before are the ones who will experience dramatic results, fast."

- Bill Phillips -

255. "Persistence can change failure into extraordinary achievement."

- Matt Biondi -

256. "If you blow your diet or skip a workout, don't get down, just pick up where you left off."

- Lee Labrada -

Planning

257. "The three factors in a good exercise program are the time you exercise, supplementation and type of exercise."

- Cory Everson -

258. "An ounce of prevention is worth a pound of cure."

- Benjamin Franklin -

259. "Schedule all of your workouts in advance; this creates accountability. Plan an entire month ahead of time. If you schedule it, you'll do it. If you wing it, you won't. It's that simple."

- Tony Horton -

260. "Pick a goal, make a realistic plan to reach that goal, work through each step of the plan, and repeat."

- Georges St. Pierre -

261. "When you combine proper nutrition with proper training the results can be staggering."

- John Christy -

262. "It's vitally important that we plan our exercise sessions in advance. They should be incorporated into your daily schedule and adhered to just as if they were an appointment at the doctor's office."

- Bill Phillips -

263. "It's not the will to win that matters — everyone has that. It's the will to prepare to win that matters."

- Paul "Bear" Bryant -

264. "Organize your eating, and eat consciously. When you don't have a plan, it's easier to give into an emotional impulse and feed haphazardly."

- Bob Greene -

265. "Things turn out best for the people who make the best of the way things turn out."

- John Wooden -

266. "Make sure your worst enemy doesn't live between your own two ears."

- Laird Hamilton -

267. "Visualization is about imagining how something relates to your senses – feel, smell, taste and sound. It's not something you just decide to do by sitting there a few minutes – like all good things, it takes practice and an open mind. But when you do it right, your imagination makes it seem so real that it can trick your body into thinking it is reality. This is a very good thing."

- Georges St. Pierre -

268. "I know how tough it can be to get to the gym, or to take your daily stroll, when all you want to do is curl up on the couch. But remember this mantra: To get energy, you need to expend it - and sooner than you think, you'll be living proof of that!"

- Denise Austin -

269. "A youthful mind is playful and lighthearted. It laughs easily, genuinely, and with abandon."

- Deepak Chopra -

270. "Giving thanks and reinforcing the positive in your life will come back to you by making you feel more positive and more motivated."

- James Beckerman -

271. "Now is the time to begin focusing on progress rather than perfection. When you do, your mindset will quickly change, and you'll gain confidence and momentum with each new day."

- Bill Phillips -

272. "Living your dream isn't about perfection. It's knowing who you are and believing anything is possible."

- Urijah Faber -

273. "Choose the positive. You have choice. You are master of your attitude. Choose the positive. The constructive. Optimism is a faith that leads to success."

- Bruce Lee -

274. "Remember, you are the mind. Your machine, your body, is at your command. Whether you want to lose 30 or 300 pounds, you can change your body. Walk it. Feed it. Water it. Rest it. Love it. Transform it."

- Chris Powell -

275. "Think and speak only positives. Do not be afraid to love yourself and what you want to become. Never, ever, allow yourself a moment of self-doubt. You must firmly believe you will become all that you desire."

- Steve Michalik -

276. "Never underestimate the power of suggestion – or your mind, for that matter. This is why it's important to weed out negative, self-defeating thoughts and replace them with positive, goal achieving thoughts."

- Lee Labrada -

277. "It does not matter how slowly you go as long as you do not stop."

- Confucius -

278. "When you increase your range of motion you not only protect yourself against injury, you also increase your body's ability to be efficient, which translates into speed for a swimmer or runner, accuracy for a tennis player, and strength for a rower or cyclist - in other words, better performance in any sport or physical activity."

- Dara Torres -

279. "Good is not good when better is expected."

- Vin Scully -

280. "Never mistake activity for achievement."

- John Wooden -

281. "To uncover your true potential you must first find your own limits and then you have to have the courage to blow past them."

- Picabo Street -

282. "Don't always train with the same amount of weight. Some days use more moderate weights to tone the muscles, on other training days really exert yourself, give the muscles plenty of work to do, then nature will take care of building more strength, muscle and better health."

- Eugene Sandow -

283. "Go slow if you must. Go easy if you must. Just go."

- Urijah Faber -

284. "Keep progressing and growing and striving. After all, that's what life is about."

- Bradley J. Steiner -

285. "Setbacks are a natural and inevitable part of any progression and are no reason to throw in the towel. If you can overcome setbacks and reach your goals in spite of them, you have shown true strength of character. Ultimately, your sense of accomplishment will be that much greater."

- Bob Greene -

286. "The cycle of life is one of continuous transformation."

- Deepak Chopra -

287. "Progress only comes in small incremental portions. Nobody becomes great overnight."

- Georges St. Pierre -

Proper Form

288. "It's very important that no matter what strength training exercises you perform, you perform them properly. At the very least, bad form while exercising can cause aches and pains, and in the worst case it can cause injury."

- Bob Greene -

289. "Always sit and stand with your back straight, stomach in and head up. Walk in the same way. When you come across a mirror, turn sideways and quickly reset your stance to reflect a perfect countenance. It will pay off."

- Jack LaLanne -

290. "Instead of responding to the urge to tell others about yourself and your accomplishments and then worry endlessly about their opinion of you, focus on them. Make it your goal to listen to the people you meet. Collect the life stories of others. Ask open-ended questions. Listen. Digest. Be present."

- Chalene Johnson -

291. "Remember this. Hold on to this. This is the only perfection there is, the perfection of helping others. This is the only thing we can do that has any lasting meaning. This is why we're here. To make each other feel safe."

- Andre Agassi -

292. "Your body is not merely a physical device that generates thoughts and feelings; rather, it is a network of energy, transformation, and intelligence in dynamic exchange with the world around you."

- Deepak Chopra -

293. "When you know someone has a tendency to be negative - even someone you might see as a rival in life - call his bluff. Give him a compliment and watch his attitude change immediately. It's powerful stuff."

- Urijah Faber -

Relaxation

294. "Meditate. Find some time when you can tune everything else out and close your eyes. Think about the path you are taking, and recognize that you are moving forward, even if it is more slowly than you might like or expect. Breathe deeply. Relax. Then open your eyes and press on."

- James Beckerman -

295. "Take a music bath once or twice a week for a few seasons, and you will find that it is to the soul what the water bath is to the body."

- Oliver Wendell Holmes -

296. "It is reasonable to conclude that an hour of sleep before midnight is worth more than an hour thereafter."

- Bernarr MacFadden -

297. "Good sleep, which I define as uninterrupted sleep for as close to eight hours as you can manage – is as important to weight loss as any of the other 'ingredients'... You need to think of it as an important component of your thin lifestyle. You can't get or stay thin long without it."

- Bob Harper -

298. "Carve out a part of your day to do nothing... In the nothingness, you'll learn more about yourself, what you need to do about who you are becoming, and what is important in your life."

- Tony Horton -

299. "Training is essential, of course, but most trainees give it exaggerated importance compared with another component of success – recuperation from training. If you don't get your recuperative system in order, you won't make good progress with your training, and muscle building."

- Stuart McRobert -

Self Improvement

300. "As simple as it sounds, we all must try to be the best person we can: by making the best choices, by making the most of the talents we've been given."

- Mary Lou Retton -

301. "Lighten up. Don't give yourself such a hard time. You don't have to be perfect... A sense of humor opens doors, releases tension, and builds new friendships and business opportunities. Run from gloom and doom, and surround yourself with happy, shiny people."

- Tony Horton -

302. "I have a friend who has a great idea about training. He says, 'You don't get better on the days when you feel like going. You get better on the days when you don't want to go, but you go anyway.'"

- Georges St. Pierre -

303. "Success is peace of mind which is a direct result of self-satisfaction in knowing you did your best to become the best you are capable of becoming."

- John Wooden -

304. "Never take good health for granted. It needs to be worked at. Take all possible actions to preserve good health – for your sake and those who depend on you."

- Stuart McRobert -

305. "Never underestimate the power of dreams and the influence of the human spirit. We are all the same in this notion: the potential for greatness lives within each of us."

- Wilma Rudolph -

306. "A man who doesn't exercise will have a weak body, a sluggish mind, weak will and will lack energy. He can hardly hope to succeed in the times that we are experiencing and can expect to continue to an uncertain time in the future. And the man that lives right and exercises right not only obtains tremendously powerful muscles that obey his every command but his internal organs perform their duties

perfectly. He also obtains a thorough mastery of his will and an easy and contented mind."

- Bob Hoffman -

307. "Exploring your identity, finding your authentic self, and getting to know your emotional side – what makes you tick and what makes you stumble – are essential for transformation. So are believing that you can do it, keeping your promises to yourself, learning to bounce back from setbacks, and surrounding yourself with people who believe in you."

- Chris Powell -

308. "The frequent employment of one's will power masters all organs of movement and trains them to perform feats which otherwise would have been difficult, painful, and even impossible. The man becomes independent and self-reliant; he will never be a coward, and, when real danger threatens, he is the one who is looked up to by others. The knowledge of one's strength entails a real mastery over oneself; it breeds energy and courage, helps one over the most difficult tasks of life, and procures contentment and true enjoyment of living."

- George Hackenschmidt -

309. "The cornerstone of all success begins with your foundation. By foundation, I mean the process of figuring out who you are, what's important to you, what gives you joy, what you want, and why you want it. When you build your life on bedrock, you stand tall, shoulders back, head up, smiling in the face of what might otherwise be a difficult decision, and just know what's right for you."

- Chalene Johnson -

310. "The rest of your life is the best of your life! So get a calendar and circle the date. The rest of your life awaits... And this is the first day."

- Jack LaLanne -

311. "You are the architect of your own body. If you can make over your body, you can make over your life."

- Denise Austin -

312. "All types of knowledge ultimately leads to self-knowledge."

- Bruce Lee -

313. "Solitary confinement is to this day, one of the harshest, legal forms of punishment that can be carried out against anyone. Unfortunately, it's one that many inflict on themselves in this modern world."

- Bill Phillips -

314. "There are 6 billion people on the planet. Pick your friends carefully."

- Chalene Johnson -

315. "Social support is the most neglected aspect of fat loss programs, but it can actually be the most important factor in your success."

- Craig Ballantyne -

316. "Keep away from people who try to belittle your ambitions. Small people always do that, but the really great make you feel that you, too, can become great."

- Mark Twain -

317. "Buddies work because buddies make you work. And vice versa. You're more likely to have success with your weight-loss plan if you involve someone else and can help make him or her successful too. People with weight loss buddies are proven to lose more weight than people who go it alone."

- James Beckerman -

318. "Everyone needs a hand once in a while, even you! When you ask for help, you show that you care about and value yourself, and have enough self-confidence to allow others to help you. By delegating, you add balance to your life, and take care of you."

- Denise Austin -

Spiritual Health

319. "The body only profits a little from exercising but the spirit profits a lot."

- Billy Blanks -

320. "You can ignore your body, but your body will never ignore you. It has faithfully taken care of you since the moment you were conceived. No matter how much you neglect or abuse it, your body doesn't abandon its mission. It exists to take care of you, if only you will let it."

- Deepak Chopra -

321. "Live for the moment, and do not harp on about what you should have been doing in former years. No matter how many mistakes you have made, no matter how much training time you have wasted, and no matter how much you wish you could turn the clock back, what is done is done."

- Stuart McRobert -

322. "Family is like a garden: You have to cultivate it. But when you do, the rewards are great. Reconnecting with or meeting with family members who live in different parts of the country can solidify your family bonds and bring back happy memories."

- Denise Austin -

323. "This is the great error of our day, that physicians separate the soul from the body. The cure should not be attempted without the treatment of the whole, and no attempt should be made to cure the body without the soul."

- Plato -

324. "Good health and good intellect are the two greatest blessings in life. If you are born with health, as most of us are, you have hope. And if you have hope you have everything."

- Jack LaLanne -

325. "The biggest fool on earth is the man who scoffs at the invincible power of the human spirit."

- Bradley J. Steiner -

326. "Only when you have self-awareness can you achieve self acceptance. Only when you accept yourself can you experience self-love. And when you're capable of self-love, you learn to love. To express love is our ultimate goal."

- Bob Greene -

Strength

327. "Being weak is a choice, so is being strong."

- Frank Zane-

328. "The fundamental principle of building a stronger body is the process of overcoming stress, or 'resistance.' We force our muscles to work, and this effort in turn forces are muscles to adapt."

- Bill Phillips -

329. "When a man is strong he has a real mastery over himself. This strength breeds energy and courage, helps to meet with success the more difficult problems and tasks of life. Results in true contentment and enjoyment of living."

- Bob Hoffman -

330. "Muscle mass does not always equal strength. Strength is kindness and sensitivity. Strength is understanding that your power is both physical and emotional. That it comes from the body and the mind. And the heart."

- Henry Rollins -

331. "It is a well known fact that the majority of men today are relatively weak, whereas the struggle for existence demands now more than at any previous epoch that we should all be strong!"

- George Hackenschmidt -

332. "The physical strength you develop will not only help you perform better in your chosen activity, but also improve the stability of your joints and the health of your bones. These benefits have far-reaching impacts on your overall lifestyle, including how active you can be with your children, how well you cope with stress from work, and even how long you will live."

- Chris Carmichael -

333. "Your desire to reach the outcome – a leaner, healthier body - must be stronger then the fear that keeps you back. There's going to be a certain amount of discomfort in approaching any goal. Your desire has to be stronger."

- Lee Labrada –

334. "Get strong. And stay strong. Workout with weights or an equivalent form of resistance training. Tune in to all your muscles. Embrace them, be proud of them, these amazing life helpers. Challenge them. Be strong enough to live to 100. Strength = life. Be as strong as you can be. You cannot be too strong."

- Walter M. Bortz II -

335. "Strength does not come from winning. Your struggles develop your strengths. When you go through hardships and decide not to surrender, that is strength."

- Arnold Schwarzenegger -

336. "There are effective ways to help protect oneself from harmful stress, and the first step is to better understand it."

- Philip Maffetone -

337. "Next time you feel emotional turbulence, immediately bring your attention to the sensations in your body and make a conscious choice to stop interpreting the emotional experience. When you have focused your attention on the bodily sensations that accompany an emotion, you have stopped all interpretation, and your mind becomes silent."

- Deepak Chopra -

338. "I believe the reason I don't have a high degree of stress is because I have kept myself busy all my life. I have tackled situations head-on rather than put myself into a state of stress with constant worry when problems arise."

- Jack LaLanne -

339. "I shall tell you a great secret, my friend. Do not wait for the last judgment, it takes place every day."

- Albert Camus -

340. "We all have time to spend or waste, and it is our decision what to do with it."

- Bruce Lee -

341. "You don't need to work out three hours a day to get results. In fact, this can lead to overtraining, boredom, and burnout. An hour a day is all you really need to make healthy, physical gains that can change your life."

- Kim Lyons -

342. "Time is too valuable to waste. Devote yourself to your job and to your family, do what you need to do, and make the time to train. If you want to train, you will find the time to train."

- Brooks Kubik -

343. "My overriding philosophy: Keep the workout short and keep it simple, and you'll stay focused and motivated."

- David Zinczenko -

344. "Ask yourself: What is 20 or 30 minutes out of my day? It's about the same amount of time it takes you to watch a television show. In that time, you could be doing something good for your body and your life. And if you can't bear to miss your favorite show, then you can even exercise while you watch it."

- Bob Greene -

345. "The accumulation of toxins in the body/mind system leads to uncontrolled weight gain, accelerated aging, and impaired physical functions. Eliminating toxins awakens the body's capacity for renewal and returning to natural balance. Toxins need to be illuminated from the body, mind, and soul."

- Deepak Chopra -

346. "Make your mind a blank so far as the past is concerned, and fill it with uplifting thoughts for the present and the future. Worry is a mental poison, the toxic element produced in the mind by retention of waste matter."

- Bernarr MacFadden -

347. "Once you conduct an honest assessment of who you are and what you can do - you have to begin to eliminate one of life's major toxins - excuses."

- Urijah Faber -

348. "Drink plenty of water to keep your body functioning properly and to wash all the toxins and impurities out of your system."

- Jack LaLanne -

Training

349. "Training is such a vital part of preparation for a game, you really do train to play. It tops up your ability, like sharpening a carving knife. You can get away with not doing it for a while, as long as you have reached a certain standard of fitness."

- Graeme Le Saux -

350. "Incorporating exercises that work on multiple planes is so crucial to achieving the strongest muscles in the least amount of time as well as the best overall fitness."

- Dara Torres -

351. "Dying is easy. Living is a pain in the butt. It's like an athletic event. You've got to train for it. You've got to eat right. You've got to exercise. Your health account, your bank account, they're the same thing. The more you put in, the more you can take out. Exercise is king and nutrition is queen: together, you have a kingdom."

- Jack LaLanne -

352. "If you train hard, you'll not only be hard, you'll be hard to beat."

- Herschel Walker -

353. "Choice of exercises and manipulation of the training variables allow each athlete to tailor the activity to individual needs and goals."

- Arnold Schwarzenegger -

354. "My philosophy is that exercise can't be like a jealous boyfriend or girlfriend - high-maintenance and more trouble than it's worth. It has to be like the perfect partner in that it complements the rest of your life. Otherwise, there's no incentive to keep to the program, and you'll just end up breaking up with it in the long run."

- David Zinczenko -

355. "I truly believe that if you want to continue getting results, you need to continually vary your workout program."

- Craig Ballantyne -

356. "We all sweat. You need to work hard enough and long enough to break a sweat. And, the better shape you are in, the more you sweat and the sooner he will begin sweating in your workout."

- Bob Greene -

357. "If you don't know where you are going, you will wind up somewhere else."

- Yogi Berra -

358. "It's the repetition of affirmations that leads to belief. Once that belief becomes a deep conviction, things begin to happen."

- Muhammad Ali -

359. "Using your imagination to create mental images stimulates your mind, helps organize your life and keeps your focus in a particular direction. It allows your unconscious mind to work toward the image your have created, the goal. It's about understanding the life you want to live, and seeing it unfold before you."

- Georges St. Pierre -

360. "Think back five years ago. Think of where you're at today. Think ahead five years about what you want to accomplish. Be unstoppable."

- Dwayne Johnson -

361. "The greatest revolution of our generation is the discovery that human beings, by changing the inner aspects of their minds, can change the outer aspects of their lives."

- William James -

362. "Never let circumstances get the better of you – you get the better of them. Get in charge and control your destiny."

- Stuart McRobert -

Walking

363. "Walking is the best possible exercise. Habituate yourself to walk very far."

- Thomas Jefferson -

364. "A vigorous five-mile walk will do more good for an unhappy but otherwise healthy adult than all the medicine and psychology in the world."

- Paul Dudley White -

365. "Don't worry if you don't feel strong at first. Most people don't, so you're not alone. It doesn't matter whether you use 100 pounds or 10 pounds for exercise. Your personal best is all that is required."

- Lee Labrada -

366. "So you want to be 'toned.' What does that mean? Well, you can't tone fat. Fat just sits there looking fat! But you can tone muscle. And how do you tone muscle? By lifting weights."

- Kim Lyons -

367. "You don't have to have some type of advanced level of fitness or some special skill before you can begin training with weights. You don't have to go through some type of special conditioning before you step into a weight room. No matter what your current level of fitness is – whether you're a beginner or you've been working out for years – if you're healthy, you are ready to step into the weight room right now."

- Bill Phillips -

368. "Your body is your responsibility. It's up to you to take care of it to the best of your abilities."

- Kim Lyons -

369. "To enjoy the glow of good health, you must exercise."

- Gene Tunney -

370. "A fit body is not necessarily a healthy body, and a healthy body is not necessarily a fit one. Fitness and health are not synonymous."

- Stuart McRobert -

371. "Time and health are two precious assets that we don't recognize and appreciate until they have been depleted."

- Denis Waitley -

372. "My experience as a school nurse taught me that we need to make a concerted effort, all of us, to increase physical fitness activity among our children and to encourage all Americans to adopt a healthier diet that includes fruits and vegetables."

- Lois Capps -

373. "Willpower has two parts; your plan and your behavior.   Solutions turn words into action."

- James Beckerman -

374. "There is a strong, lean body inside you, and you have the power to release it."

- Lee Labrada -

375. "Lots of people ask me whether they can become strong.   Most certainly!   You all can acquire great strength, if you have the will and proper guidance.   But before all, you must cultivate will power, and this first lesson is the most important one.   If physical exercises alone, without your will and mind, were all that was needful, everyone could become a strong man, whether he be a brain or muscle worker."

- George Hackenschimdt -

376. "When you slow down too much, you come to a stop."

- Jack LaLanne -

377. "Strength does not come from physical capacity. It comes from an indomitable will."

- Bruce Lee -

378. "Resilience is going to pay off."

- Cat Zingano -

379. "A will is to make a decision how you should take care of yourself."

- Billy Blanks -

Biographies

Agassi, Andre

Occupation: Professional Tennis Player &
Philanthropist.

Known for: Agassi won the Grand Slam
Championship in tennis 8-times. Along with
winning many other tennis championships, Agassi
also won a gold medal in the 1996 Olympics for
tennis.

Published works include: 'Open: An
Autobiography.'

Ali, Muhammad

Occupation: Professional Boxer.

Known for: Becoming World Heavyweight
Champion at age 22, Ali had 31 wins as a boxer
before suffering his first loss at the hands of Joe
Frazier, who he came back to beat a few years later
in New York City.

Published works include: 'Soul of a Butterfly:
Reflections on Life's Journey.'

Aristotle

Occupation: Ancient Greek Philosopher &
Scientist.

Known for: Aristotle was a pupil of Plato and Tutor to Alexander the Great.

Published works include: 'Corpus Aristotelicum.'

Austin, Denise

Occupation: Fitness Instructor, Author & Columnist.

Known for: Besides producing numerous videos and books on fitness, Austin has also served as a past member of the U.S. President's Council on Physical Fitness & Sports.

Published works include: 'Fit and Fabulous after 40' & 'Get Energy!: Empower Your Body, Love Your Life.'

Ballantyne, Craig

Occupation: Fitness Instructor & Author.

Known for: Ballantyne is the founder of the Turbulence Training Fitness System.

Published works include: 'The Ultimate Guide to TT Metabolic Resistance Training', 'Turbulence Training for Fat Loss' & 'Just Say No to Cardio.'

Baroni, Bill

Occupation: Law Professor & Former New Jersey State Senator.

Published works include: 'Fat Kid Got Fit: And So Can You!'

Beckerman, James

Occupation: Medical Doctor & Cardiologist.

Known for: Beckerman has served as the chair of the Oregon Governor's Council on Physical Fitness & Sports.

Published works include: 'The Flex Diet: Design-Your-Own Weight Loss Plan.'

Berra, Yogi

Occupation: Former Major League Baseball Catcher, Manager & Coach.

Known for: Along with winning 13 World Series and numerous other distinctions, Berra was elected to the Baseball Hall of Fame in 1972.

Published works include: 'When You Come to a Fork in the Road, Take It!', 'What Time Is It? You Mean Now?: Advice for Life from the Zennest Master of Them All' & 'The Yogi Book.'

Bhave, Vinoba

Occupation: Human Rights Advocate & Indian Advocate of Nonviolence.

Published works include: 'Moved by Love: The Memoirs of Vinoba Bhave.'

Billings, Josh

Occupation: 19th Century Humor Writer & Lecturer.

Published works include: 'The Compete Works of Josh Billings.'

Biondi, Matt
Occupation: Former Champion Swimmer & Educator.
Known for: Biondi has won a total of 11 Olympic Medals and is a former world-record holder in five events.

Blanchard, Rachel
Occupation: Actress.
Known for: Blanchard has appeared in numerous television & film roles including 'Snakes on a Plane,' '7ᵗʰ Heaven' & 'The Case for Christmas.'

Blanks, Billy
Occupation: Fitness Instructor, Martial Artist & Actor.
Known for: Blanks is the founder of the Tae Bo exercise system.
Published works include: 'The Tae Bo Way.'

Bortz II, Walter M.
Occupation: Educator & Higher Education Administrator.
Published works include: 'The Roadmap to 100: The Breakthrough Science of Living a Long and Healthy Life.'

Bryant, Paul "Bear"

Occupation: College American Football Coach.

Known for: Bryant took the University of Alabama football team to six national championship wins and thirteen conference championship victories.

Published works include: 'Bear: The Hard Life and Good Times of Alabama's Coach Bryant.'

Camus, Albert

Occupation: Writer & Philosopher.

Known for: Camus contributed to the rise of the philosophy known as Absurdism.

Published works include: 'Betwixt and Between' & 'The Stranger.'

Capps, Lois

Occupation: Politician, Nurse & College Professor.

Known for: Capps has been a California Representative in the US House of Representatives since 1998.

Carano, Gina

Occupation: Professional Mixed Martial Arts Fighter & Actress.

Known for: Aside from building a reputation as a pioneer in women's mixed martial arts, Carano has appeared in films 'Haywire' and 'Fast & Furious 6'

along with a stint as the gladiator Crush on NBC's
television series 'American Gladiators.'

Carmichael, Chris

Occupation: Cyclist & Coach.

Known for: Carmichael competed in the Tour de
France & the 1984 Summer Olympics.

Published works include: 'Chris Carmichael's Food
for Fitness: Eat Right to Train Right' & '5
Essentials for a Winning Life: The Nutrition,
Fitness, and Life Plan for Discovering the
Champion Within.'

Chopra, Deepak

Occupation: Physician, Alternative Medicine
Advocate, Speaker & Writer.

Known for: Chopra appeared on 'The Oprah
Winfrey Show' to explain many of his findings and
became a leading advocate of the 'mind-body'
connection.

Published works include: 'Perfect Health', 'What
are you Hungry for?' & 'Grow Younger, Live
Longer.'

Christy, John

Occupation: Strength Coach & Writer.

Published works include: 'Real Strength, Real
Muscle.'

Churchill, Winston

Occupation: British Prime Minister, Historian & Writer.

Known for: Churchill served many years in the British government and lead and inspired the British people through their most difficult conflict with Germany in World War II.

Published works include: 'My Early Life: 1874 - 1904', 'Memoirs of the Second World War' & 'Never Give In! The Best of Winston Churchill's Speeches.'

Confucius

Occupation: Ancient Chinese Philosopher, Teacher & Politician.

Known for: Confucius's teachings and writings formed a well-known philosophical system known as 'Confucianism.'

Published works include: 'The Five Classics.'

Cool J, LL

Occupation: Hip Hop Entertainer, Actor & Entrepreneur.

Known for: LL Cool J has had numerous Top 40 hits on American radio and acting in films such as 'Halloween H20' & 'Deep Blue Sea.'

Published works include: 'I Make My Own Rules' & 'LL Cool J's Platinum 360 Diet and Lifestyle: A

Full-Circle Guide to Developing Your Mind, Body and Soul.'

Cooper, Jay
Occupation: Director of Wellness at Green Valley Spa in St. George, Utah.

Published works include: 'Body Code.'

Doherty, Ken
Occupation: Professional Snooker Player & BBC Radio Commentator.

Known for: At the time of publication, Doherty is the only player to have been a world amateur and world professional champion snooker player.

Published works include: 'Ken Doherty: Life in the Frame: My Story.'

Dorsett, Tony
Occupation: Professional American Football Player.

Known for: Dorsett played running back for the National Football League teams the Dallas Cowboys and the Denver Broncos.

Published works include: 'Running Tough: Memoirs of a Football Maverick.'

Durant, Will
Occupation: Historian, Philosopher & Writer.

Known for: Durant wrote 11 volumes of a series of books called 'The Story of Civilization.'

Published works include: 'The Story of Civilization' & 'The Story of Philosophy.'

Einstein, Albert

Occupation: Theoretical Physicist & Scientific Philosopher.

Known for: Einstein developed and published hundreds of scientific and non-scientific works. In popular culture, he is credited with the development of the theory of relativity.

Published works include: 'The World As I See It', 'Ideas and Opinions' & 'Relativity: The Special and General Theory.'

Everson, Cory

Occupation: Female Bodybuilder, Actress & Fitness Instructor.

Known for: Everson is a 6-time consecutive Ms. Olympia Champion.

Published works include: 'Cory Everson's Fat-Free & Fit' & 'Cory Everson's Life Balance.'

Faber, Urijah

Occupation: Professional Mixed Martial Arts Fighter.

Known for: Faber is a former World Extreme Cage Fighting Bantamweight Champion and UFC title contender.

Published works include: 'The Laws of the Ring: The Laws of the Cage from the California Kid.'

Franklin, Benjamin

Occupation: Author, Politician, Philosopher, Postmaster & American Statesman.

Known for: Franklin was instrumental in the bringing forth of numerous inventions & scientific contributions. He also spent many years overseas as an ambassador for the United States in France during the War of Independence from Great Britain.

Published works include: 'The Autobiography of Benjamin Franklin' & 'Poor Richard's Almanac.'

Greene, Bob

Occupation: Personal Trainer, Author & Entrepreneur.

Known for: Greene was instrumental in helping talk show host, Oprah Winfrey, lose a considerable amount of weight along with helping her prepare to successfully run a marathon.

Published works include: 'Make the Connection: Ten Steps to a Better Body and a Better Life', 'Get with the Program!: Getting Real about your

Weight, Health, and Emotional Well-Being', &
'Best Life Diet.'

Hackenschmidt, George

Occupation: Early 20ᵗʰ Century Strongman,
Writer & Philosopher.

Known for: Hackenschmidt not only performed
many public feats of strength, he also was a well
known professional wrestler whom many credit
with creating the move, the 'bear hug.'

Published works include: 'The Way to Live' &
'Complete Science of Wrestling.'

Halas, George

Occupation: Football Player, Coach & Team
Owner.

Known for: Halas is best know for founding the
Chicago Bears.

Published works include: 'Halas by Halas: The
Autobiography of George Halas.'

Hamilton, Bethany

Occupation: Professional Surfer.

Known for: Hamilton survived a 2003 shark
attack that left her with one arm, but she returned
to professional surfing and has won or placed near
the top in numerous competitions.

Published works include: 'Soul Surfer: A True Story of Faith, Family, and Fighting to Get Back on the Board.'

Hamilton, Laird
Occupation: Professional Surfer & Model.
Published works include: 'Force of Nature: Mind, Body, Soul, and, Of Course, Surfing.'

Haney, Lee
Occupation: Professional Bodybuilder.
Known for: Haney is best known for tying for a record IFBB Mr. Olympia wins at 8. He has also served as the Chairman of the US President's Council on Physical Fitness & Sports.
Published works include: 'Totalee Awesome: A Complete Guide to Body-Building Success' & 'Lee Haney's Ultimate Bodybuilding.'

Harper, Bob
Occupation: TV Personality, Personal Trainer & Author.
Known for: Harper was one of the first trainers featured in the popular US television show 'The Biggest Loser.'
Published works include: 'Are You Ready!: Take Charge, Lose Weight, Get in Shape, and Change' & 'Skinny Meals: Everything You Need to Lose Weight-Fast!'

<u>Hippocrates</u>

Occupation: Ancient Greek Philosopher.

Known for: Often credited with being the 'father of western medicine.'

Published works include: 'Works of Hippocrates.'

<u>Hoffman, Bob</u>

Occupation: Magazine Publisher, US Olympic Weightlifting Coach & Physical Culturalist.

Known for: Hoffman has been called The 'Father of World Weightlifting' and also was the founder of the York Barbell Club.

Published works include: 'How to be Strong, Healthy and Happy' & 'Bob Hoffman's Simplified System of Barbell Training.'

<u>Holmes, Oliver Wendell</u>

Occupation: US Supreme Court Justice.

Known for: Holmes was a long-serving United States Supreme Court Justice.

Published works include: 'The Essential Holmes' & 'The Autocrat of the Breakfast Table.'

<u>Holtz, Lou</u>

Occupation: College American Football Coach & Television Personality.

Known for: Holtz coached football at numerous American universities leading many to national victories.

Published works include: 'Winning Every Day' & 'Wins, Losses, and Lessons.'

Holyfield, Evander
Occupation: Professional Boxer.
Known for: Holyfield is known to be the only 4-time World Heavyweight Champion in boxing at time of publication.
Published works include: 'Becoming Holyfield: A Fighter's Journey.'

Horton, Tony
Occupation: Fitness Instructor.
Known for: Horton is the founder of the P90X Fitness System.
Published works include: 'Bring It!' & 'Crush It!'

Hubbard, Elbert
Occupation: Writer & Publisher.
Known for: Hubbard was a founder of the Roycroft artisan community in New York.
Published works include: 'Little Journeys to the Homes of Good Men and Great' & 'Health & Wealth.'

Inch, Thomas
Occupation: Professional Strong Man.
Known for: For a time, Inch held the title of 'Britain's Strongest Man.'

Published works include: 'On Strength.'

<u>Jackson, Bo</u>

Occupation: Professional American Football & Baseball Player.

Known for: At time of publication, Jackson was named 'Greatest Athlete of All Time' by ESPN. Also, Jackson appeared in numerous Nike advertisements in the late 1980s.

Published works include: 'Bo Knows Bo.'

<u>Jackson, Phil</u>

Occupation: Professional Basketball Player & Coach.

Known for: While a respectable player for the New York Knicks and then the New Jersey Nets during his playing career, Jackson coached the Chicago Bulls to six National Basketball Championships and the Los Angeles Lakers to five. He was also inducted into the Naismith Memorial Basketball Hall of Fame.

Published works include: 'Eleven Rings: The Soul of Success' & 'Sacred Hoops: Spiritual Lessons of a Hardwood Warrior.'

<u>James, William</u>

Occupation: Psychologist & Philosopher.

Known for: It has been said that James was a leader in late 19[a] Century psychology. He's been called 'The Father of American psychology.' He was the first educator to offer a course on psychology in the United States.

Published works include: 'The Principles of Psychology' & 'Pragmatism.'

Jefferson, Thomas

Occupation: U.S. President, Ambassador & Inventor.

Known for: A Founding Father of the United States and primary author of the Declaration of Independence, Jefferson served as the third President of the United States of America.

Published works include: 'Thomas Jefferson: Writings: (Library of America #17).'

Johnson, Chalene

Occupation: Physical Fitness Instructor & Writer.

Known for: Johnson is credited with creating the exercise systems 'TurboJam' & 'TurboFire.'

Published works include: 'PUSH: 30 Days to Turbocharged Habits, a Bangin' Body, and the Life You Deserve!'

Johnson, Dwayne

Occupation: Professional Wrestler, Actor & Producer.

Known for: One of the most charismatic performers in Hollywood, Johnson began his entertainment career as a professional wrestler known as "The Rock." He has appeared in numerous films which include 'Fast Five', 'The Other Guys', 'Get Smart' & 'Walking Tall' to name a few.

Jordan, Michael

Occupation: Professional Basketball Player & Basketball Team Owner.

Known for: Jordan led the Chicago Bulls basketball team to six total NBA Championships.

Published works include: 'I Can't Accept Not Trying' & 'For the Love of the Game: My Story.'

Joyner-Kersee, Jackie

Occupation: Olympic Track and Field Athlete.

Known for: Joyner-Kersey won 3 Olympic gold medals along with being voted the Greatest Female Athlete of the 20th Century by 'Sports Illustrated for Women' Magazine.

Published works include: 'A Kind of Grace: The Autobiography of the World's Greatest Female Athlete.'

Joyner, Florence Griffith

Occupation: Olympic Track and Field Athlete.

Known for: Joyner 3 Olympic gold medals in the 1988 Seoul Olympics.

Kaehler, Kathy

Occupation: Personal Trainer & Author.

Known for: Koehler has had a lengthy career of training numerous celebrities such as Julia Roberts, Cindy Crawford, Jennifer Anniston and many others.

Published works include: 'Kathy Koehler's Celebrity Workouts: How to get a Hollywood Body in Just 30 Minutes a Day' & 'Fit & Sexy for Life.'

Kennedy, John F.

Occupation: US President.

Known for: Kennedy was the 35ᵗ President of the United States. During his term as president, he oversaw the initiation of Project Apollo (the space program) and the Cuban Missile Crisis.

Published works include: 'Profiles in Courage.'

Kiam, Victor

Occupation: Entrepreneur & American Football Team Owner.

Known for: Kiam purchased Remington Products and became Chief Executive Office and Spokesman for the company. Kiam went on to become the owner of the New England Patriots Football Team.

Published works include: 'Go for It! How to Succeed as an Entrepreneur' & 'Live to Win: Achieving Success in Life and Business.'

Knight, Bobby
Occupation: College & Olympic Team Basketball Coach.

Known for: A controversial figure in collegiate sports, Knight's accomplishments include coaching the 1984 US men's Olympic basketball team to a gold medal and winning numerous NCAA championship games while coaching for the Indiana University Hoosiers.

Published works include: 'Knight: My Story.'

Korbut, Olga
Occupation: Gymnast.

Known for: Soviet-born Korbut won numerous gold medals in gymnastics for the Soviet Union at the 1972 Summer Olympics in Munich, Germany.

Kubik, Brooks
Occupation: Attorney & Writer.

Known for: Kubik is a five-time national bench press champion along with being credited as a founder of the "Dinosaur Training" philosophy.

Published works include: 'Dinosaur Training' & 'Dinosaur Bodyweight Training.'

Labrada, Lee

Occupation: Professional Bodybuilder & Entrepreneur.

Known for: A winner of many national bodybuilding championships, Labrada was a regular appearance and high place finisher at numerous Mr. Olympia contests from the late-1980s into the mid-1990s.

Published works include: 'The Lean Body Promise. Burn Away Fat and Release the Leaner, Stronger Body Inside You.'

LaLanne, Jack

Occupation: Fitness Instructor, Writer, Entrepreneur & TV Personality.

Known for: LaLanne accomplished many physical feats during his lifetime which included swimming the length of the Golden Gate Bridge more than once while shackled and towing different types of vessels over that distance. He also is credited with setting a world record of performing 1033 push-ups in 23 minutes on a national television program. A one-time national television personality, LaLanne also is said to have beaten champion bodybuilder Arnold

Schwarzenegger in an informal contest of who could perform the most chin-ups.

Published works include: 'Live Young Forever', 'The Jack LaLanne Way to Vibrant Good Health' & 'Revitalize Your Life.'

Le Saux, Graeme

Occupation: European Football Player.

Known for: Le Saux was twice named in the Professional Footballers' Association Team of the Year, in 1995 and in 1998.

Published works include: 'Graeme Le Saux: Left Field: A Footballer Apart.'

Lee, Bruce

Occupation: Martial Artist, Actor & Philosopher.

Known for: Though he passed away unexpectedly at a young age, Lee had a prolific film and television career in the late 1960s into the early 1970s. Lee was the founder of the martial art Jeet Kune Do.

Published works include: 'Chinese Gung Fu: The Philosophical Art of Self Defense' & 'Tao of Jeet Kune Do.'

Lincoln, Abraham

Occupation: US President.

Known for: Lincoln was the 16th President of the United States of America.

Published works include: 'Speeches & Letters of Abraham Lincoln.'

Lombardi, Vince

Occupation: American Football Player & Coach.

Known for: As head coach of the Green Bay Packers, Lombardi led his team to 3 straight and 5 total National Football League championships over the course of 7 years. This total includes winning the first two Super Bowls in the mid-1960s. Lombardi is also regarded as one of the first NFL coaches to ignore the prejudices associated with racism in professional football.

Published works include: 'Run to Daylight.'

Lyons, Kim

Occupation: Personal Trainer, Television Personality & Fitness Model.

Known for: Lyons is probably best known as appearing as one of the trainers on the popular American television program 'The Biggest Loser.'

Published works include: 'Kim Lyons: Your Body, Your Life.'

MacFadden, Bernarr

Occupation: Physical Culturalist & Magazine Publisher.

Known for: An advocate for health, fitness & good nutrition, Macfadden was very influential in the early-20th Century development of physical culture.

Published works include: 'Physical Training', 'Strength from Eating' & 'Making Old Bodies Young.'

Maffetone, Philip

Occupation: Doctor & Writer.

Known for: Maffetone has developed a reputation as one of the leading trainers of endurance athletes.

Published works include: 'The Big Book of Health and Fitness' & 'The Big Book of Endurance Training and Racing.'

Maldonado, Pastor

Occupation: Race Car Driver.

Known for: Maldonado is the first Venezuelan to win a Formula One Grand Prix.

McRobert, Stuart

Occupation: Writer, Publisher & Educator.

Known for: McRobert is best known for establishing and running the independent strength training magazine 'Hardgainer.'

Published works include: 'Brawn', 'Beyond Brawn' & 'Build Muscle, Lose Fat, Look Great.'

Michaels, Jillian

Occupation: Personal Trainer & Television Personality.

Known for: Michaels has appeared on numerous television programs, most notably as a trainer on the inaugural season of the popular American television series 'The Biggest Loser.'

Published works include: 'Unlimited: How to Build an Exceptional Life' & 'Making the Cut: The 30-Day Diet and Fitness Plan for the Strongest, Sexiest You.'

Michalik, Steve

Occupation: Bodybuilder.

Known for: One of the few men who completed what has been called the 'Triple-Crown of Bodybuilding Championships' by winning the Mr. America, Mr. Universe and Mr. USA competitions.

Published works include: 'Atomic Fitness.'

Mowry, Tia

Occupation: Actress.

Known for: Mowry starred on the television series 'Sister, Sister' with her twin Tamera. Since that time, she has also starred on the Nickelodeon television show 'Instant Mom.'

Published works include: 'Oh, Baby! Pregnancy Tales and Advice from One Hot Mama to Another.'

Namath, Joe
Occupation: American Football Player.

Known for: Namath is a popular professional football quarterback who most notably played for the NFL team the New York Jets.

Norris, Chuck
Occupation: Martial Artist & Actor.

Known for: Despite a resurgence in popularity in recent years thanks to many jokes proclaiming his invincibility, Norris has starred in numerous action films and the long-running television series 'Walker, Texas Ranger.'

Published works include: 'Against All Odds: My Story' & 'The Secret Power Within.'

Otto, Jim
Occupation: Professional American Football Player.

Known for: Otto was best known for playing center for the Oakland Raiders in the 1960s and 1970s.

Published works include: 'Jim Otto: The Pain of Glory.'

Owens, Jesse

Occupation: Track & Field Athlete.

Known for: Owens was a multiple gold medalist in the 1936 Summer Olympic Games in Berlin.

Published works include: 'Jesse: The Man who Outran Hitler' & 'Track and Field.'

Oz, Daphne

Occupation: Television Personality.

Published works include: 'The Dorm Room Diet: The 10-Step Program for Creating a Healthy Lifestyle That Really Works' & 'Relish: An Adventure in Food, Style, and Everyday Fun.'

Paine, Thomas

Occupation: Philosopher, Pamphleteer & Political Activist.

Known for: Paine was instrumental in influencing the thinking of many American colonists to begin the fight for independence from Great Britain when he wrote the pamphlet 'Common Sense.'

Published works include: 'Rights of Man' & 'The Age of Reason.'

Palmer, Arnold

Occupation: Professional Golfer.

Known for: During his long professional golf career, Palmer amassed many wins which included seven major championships.

Published works include: 'A Golfer's Life' & '495 Golf Lessons.'

Patton, George S.

Occupation: US Army General.

Known for: Patton was an instrumental leader of American troops in both the First and Second World Wars. He also competed in the 1912 Modern Olympic Pentathlon - the first modern Olympic Games.

Published works include: 'War as I Knew It.'

Phillips, Bill

Occupation: Writer & Publisher.

Known for: Phillips is probably best known for establishing the popular 'Body-for-Life' body transformation program where participants submit before and after pictures and essays of their transformations from sedentary lifestyles to healthier ones. Phillips also published the once popular 'Muscle Media' magazine.

Published works include: 'Body for Life: 12 Weeks to Mental and Physical Strength' & 'Transformation.'

Plato

Occupation: Ancient Greek Philosopher.

Known for: Plato is considered one of the most influential early thinkers of Western thought and philosophy.

Published works include: 'The Republic' & 'Plato: Complete Works.'

Powell, Chris

Occupation: Personal Trainer & Television Personality.

Known for: Powell is probably best known for appearing on the ABC television series 'Extreme Weight Loss.' He has also appeared on many other shows such as '20/20' and 'Good Morning America.'

Published works include: 'Choose to Lose: The 7-Day Carb Cycle Solution.'

Rath, Tom

Occupation: Writer & Speaker.

Known for: Rath has written books that have appeared hundreds of times on the Wall Street Journal bestseller list.

Published works include: 'Strengths Based Leadership' & 'Eat Move Sleep: How Small Choices Lead to Big Changes.'

Reinagel, Monica

Occupation: Nutritionist.

Known for: Reinagel hosts the 'Nutrition Diva' podcast. She has made numerous television appearances.

Published works include: 'Nutrition Diva's Secrets for a Healthy Diet' & 'The Inflammation-Free Diet Plan.'

Retton, Mary Lou

Occupation: US Olympic Gymnast and member of the US President's Council on Physical Fitness and Sports.

Known for: Retton won a gold medal for the United States at the 1984 Summer Olympics for gymnastics.

Published works include: 'Mary Lou: Creating an Olympic Champion' & 'Mary Lou Retton's Gateways to Happiness.'

Riley, Pat

Occupation: Professional Basketball Player & Coach.

Known for: Head coach of the Los Angeles Lakers, New York Knicks and the Miami Heat, Riley has led professional NBA teams to five NBA Championships.

Published works include: 'The Winner Within: A Life Plan for Team Players.'

Rohn, Jim

Occupation: Writer, Speaker & Entrepreneur.

Known for: Rohn is considered a pioneer of the personal development and self-improvement movement in the 20th Century.

Published works include: 'Five Major Pieces to the Life Puzzle.'

Rollins, Henry

Occupation: Musician, Writer & Actor.

Known for: Rollins was the frontman for the hardcore punk band 'Black Flag' in the 1980s. He also has appeared in films such as 'Heat' and 'Bad Boys II.'

Published works include: 'The Portable Henry Rollins.'

Rousey, Ronda

Occupation: Professional Mixed Martial Artist & Actress.

Known for: Rousey is the first woman to hold a title in the professional mixed martial arts organization, the UFC. She was the first UFC Women's Bantamweight Champion. Prior to fighting in mixed martial arts, Rousey was an accomplished Judoist winning a bronze medal for the United States in the 2008 Summer Olympics.

Published works include: 'My Fight/Your Fight.'

Rudolph, Wilma

Occupation: Track & Field Athlete.

Known for: Rudolph may be best known for being the first American woman to win 3 gold medals in the 1960 Summer Olympics in Rome, Italy.

Sallis, Robert

Occupation: Medical Doctor.

Known for: Dr. Sallis is a major advocate of walking and promoting general, regular physical activity.

Published works include: 'Sports Medicine: Just the Facts.'

Salo, Mikko

Occupation: Athlete.

Known for: Salo is the winner of the 2009 CrossFit Games.

Sandow, Eugene

Occupation: Physical Culturalist & Professional Strongman.

Known for: Sandow was an early advocate of health and fitness in the early 20ᵗʰ Century. He is credited as being one of the first strongmen who combine physical symmetry with functional strength and athleticism.

Published works include: 'Strength and How to Obtain It' & 'Sandow's System of Physical Training.'

Sansone, Leslie

Occupation: Fitness Instructor & Writer.

Known for: Samson has been an advocate of health and fitness for many years, primarily promoting walking as exercise.

Published works include: 'Leslie Sansone: Walk Away the Pounds.'

Schilling, Taylor

Occupation: Actress.

Known for: Schilling stars in the Netflix original series 'Orange Is The New Black.'

Schwarzenegger, Arnold

Occupation: Film Actor, Writer, Bodybuilder & Politician.

Known for: Schwarzenegger's rise to fame began in the 1960s as he became an international bodybuilding champion winning a total of seven IFBB Mr. Olympia titles. Schwarzenegger then continued into the 1980s starring in numerous blockbuster films such as 'Commando', 'The Terminator', 'Predator' and many others. After a long, prolific acting career, Schwarzenegger then served as governor of California for two terms.

Published works include: 'The New Encyclopedia of Modern Bodybuilding' & 'Arnold's Bodybuilding for Men.'

Scully, Vin

Occupation: Sports Broadcaster.

Known for: Scully holds the record of having the longest tenure as the play-by-play announcer with a professional baseball team, the Los Angeles Dodgers.

Published works include: 'The Dodgers: From Coast to Coast.'

Seneca the Younger

Occupation: Ancient Roman Philosopher.

Known for: Seneca is one of the few popular Roman philosophers of his time.

Published works include: 'Stoic Philosophy of Seneca: Essays and Letters.'

Sidney, Phillip

Occupation: Poet & Soldier.

Known for: A prolific writer, Sir Sidney died a the young age of 31, after being injured in combat.

Published works include: 'Sir Phillip Sidney: The Major Works.'

Silva, Anderson

Occupation: Professional Mixed Martial Artist.

Known for: Regarded by many as one of the greatest mixed martial artists of all time, at time of publication, Silva holds the longest-running title defense streak in UFC history with a total 16 consecutive wins and 10 title defenses.

Published works include: 'The Mixed Martial Arts Instruction Manual: Striking.'

St. Augustine

Occupation: Philosopher & Christian Theologian.

Known for: Augustine of Hippo is considered by some to be a major influence on the development of Western Christianity and Western Philosophy.

Published works include: 'Confessions' & 'City of God.'

St. Pierre, Georges

Occupation: Professional Mixed Martial Arts Fighter & Actor.

Known for: St. Pierre was the reigning welterweight champion in the UFC with the most successful welterweight title defenses at a total of 9 at time of publication.

Published works include: 'The Way of the Fight.'

Stanhope, Philip

Occupation: British Statesman.

Published works include: 'Letters to His Son on the Art of Becoming a Man of the World and a Gentleman.'

Steiner, Bradley J.
Occupation: Writer.
Published works include: 'Powerlifting and the Development of Herculean Super-Strength.'

Stosur, Samantha
Occupation: Professional Tennis Player.
Known for: Stosur has won multiple Grand Slam titles in both singles and women's doubles events. She was also ranked first in the world for doubles.

Strachan, Gordon
Occupation: European Football Player & Manager.
Known for: After a long, successful career as a midfielder in European football (soccer), Strachan went on to manage numerous football teams. He is also a member of the Scottish Football Hall of Fame.
Published works include: 'Strachan: My Life in Football.'

Street, Picabo
Occupation: Professional Downhill Skier.

Known for: Street won a silver medal in the 1994 Winter Olympics and then went on to win the gold in the 1998 Winter Olympics.

Published works include: 'Picabo: Nothing to Hide.'

Thicke, Alan

Occupation: Television Actor & Television Game Show Host.

Known for: Thicke is best known for portraying dad, Jason Seaver on the popular 1980s sitcom 'Growing Pains.'

Published works include: 'How to Raise Kids Who Won't Hate You: Bringing Up Rockstars and Other Forms of Children.'

Thorne-Smith, Courtney

Occupation: Actress.

Known for: Smith is most well-known for her roles in American television series such as 'Ally McBeal' and 'According to Jim.'

Tolstoy, Leo

Occupation: Novelist & Philosopher.

Known for: Considered by many to be one of the giants of Russian literature, Tolstoy's most popular novels include 'Anna Karenina' and 'War and Peace.'

Torres, Dara

Occupation: Swimmer.

Known for: Torres has competed in 5 Summer Olympic Games spanning from 1984 to 2008. She has won a total of 4 gold medals in the Olympics and has always won at least one medal for each of the 5 games in which she participated.

Published works include: 'Age is Just a Number: Achieve Your Dreams at Any Stage in your Life' & 'Gold Medal Fitness.'

Tunney, Gene

Occupation: Professional Boxer.

Known for: Tunney was World Heavyweight Boxing Champion from 1926 to 1928, defeating boxing great Jack Dempsey twice.

Published works include: 'A Man Must Fight.'

Twain, Mark

Occupation: Humorist & Writer.

Known for: Some of Twain's most popular fictional works include 'The Adventures of Tom Sawyer' and 'Adventures of Huckleberry Finn.'

von Humboldt, Wilhelm

Occupation: Philosopher & Diplomat.

Known for: Founder of the Prussian education system.

Waitley, Denis
Occupation: Motivational Speaker & Consultant.
Published works include: 'The Psychology of Winning' & 'Quantum Fitness: Breakthrough to Excellence.'

Walker, Herschel
Occupation: Professional American Football Player.
Known for: An all-around athlete, Walker has not only competed extensively in football, but also had a successful, but short-lived career in mixed martial arts competition.
Published works include: 'Herschel Walker's Basic Training.'

Walsh, Kerri
Occupation: Professional Beach Volleyball Player.
Known for: Walsh and her long time teammate, Misty May-Treanor have won numerous world championships and 3 gold medals at the 2004, 2008 and 2012 Summer Olympics.

Ward, William A.
Occupation: Writer.

Known for: Ward has been called 'one of America's most quoted writers of inspirational maxims.'

Published works include: 'Thoughts of a Christian Optimist' & 'Fountains of Faith.'

Weider, Ben

Occupation: Bodybuilding Advocate & Entrepreneur.

Known for: Weider, along with his brother Joe, worked to promote the activity of competitive bodybuilding throughout the world. He was also a published expert on the history of Napoleon Bonaparte.

Published works include: 'Superpump!: Hardcore Women's Bodybuilding.'

Weider, Joe

Occupation: Magazine Publisher and Fitness Advocate.

Known for: Weider, along with his brother Ben, co-founded the International Federation of Bodybuilders. He was also the publisher of numerous fitness magazines such as 'Muscle & Fitness', 'Shape' & 'Men's Fitness.'

Published works include: 'Joe Weider's Bodybuilding System.'

White, Paul Dudley

Occupation: Cardiologist.

Known for: White was the leading cardiologist of his day and a well-known advocate of preventative medicine.

Published works include: 'My Life and Medicine: An autobiographical memoir.'

Winfrey, Oprah

Occupation: Television Talk Show Host, Media Mogul and Philanthropist.

Known for: Oprah's best-known achievement was her long-running, multiple-award-winning nationally syndicated talk show.

Published works include: 'What I know for Sure.'

Wooden, John

Occupation: Collegiate Basketball Player & Coach.

Known for: While accomplished as a collegiate player, Wooden's greatest achievement may be coaching UCLA's basketball team to 10 NCAA national championships in a 12-year period.

Published works include: 'Wooden: A Lifetime of Observations and Reflections On and Off the Court.'

Yamaguchi, Kristi

Occupation: Professional Figure Skater.

Known for: Yamaguchi competed in and won many international skating competitions, but will likely be best remembered for winning a gold medal at the 1992 Winter Olympics.

Published works include: 'Always Dream (Positively for Kids)'

Zane, Frank

Occupation: Professional Bodybuilder & Teacher.

Known for: Known for his distinctive symmetry as a physique competitor, Zane is a 3-time Mr. Olympia winner. He is also said to be one of only three men to ever beat Arnold Schwarzenegger in bodybuilding competition.

Published works include: 'The Mind in Bodybuilding', 'The High Def Handbook' & 'Frank Zane Training Manual.'

Zinczenko, David

Occupation: Author & Entrepreneur.

Known for: Zinczenko has written for publications such as 'Men's Journal' and 'Men's Fitness.'

Published works include: 'Eat This, Not That!' & 'The Abs Diet.'

Zingano, Cat

Occupation: Professional Mixed Martial Arts Fighter.

Known for: Zingano became the first woman to win a UFC fight by technical knockout against fellow competitor Miesha Tate.

About the Author

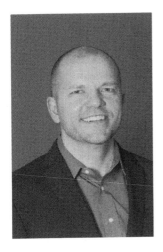

Cameron M. Clark has practiced a balanced, healthy approach to life and well-being for over two decades. He holds a Bachelor's of Science in Communications from Southern Utah University. He is also a formerly-certified personal trainer with the American Council on Exercise. Currently, Cameron is the part owner of a locally-owned professional services company in Las Vegas, Nevada. He and his wife are the parents of three children.

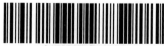

Made in the USA
San Bernardino, CA
11 July 2018